# DON'T EAT THIS IF YOU'RE TAKING THAT

## THE HIDDEN RISKS OF MIXING FOOD AND MEDICINE

Madelyn Fernstrom, PhD, CNS
and John Fernstrom, PhD

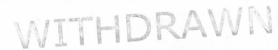

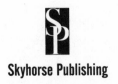
Skyhorse Publishing

Skyhorse Publishing books may be purchased in bulk at special discounts for sales promotion, corporate gifts, fund-raising, or educational purposes. Special editions can also be created to specifications. For details, contact the Special Sales Department, Skyhorse Publishing, 307 West 36th Street, 11th Floor, New York, NY 10018 or info@skyhorsepublishing.com.

Skyhorse® and Skyhorse Publishing® are registered trademarks of Skyhorse Publishing, Inc.®, a Delaware corporation.

Visit our website at www.skyhorsepublishing.com.

10 9 8 7 6 5 4 3 2 1

Library of Congress Cataloging-in-Publication Data is available on file.

Cover design by Georgia Morrissey
Cover photographs: Thinkstock

ISBN: 978-1-63220-452-3
Ebook ISBN: 978-1-63220-925-2

Printed in the United States of America

In loving memory of Emanuel M. Hirsch

# Contents

# Introduction

Our interest in food and medicine interactions began at home, with our own family. As neuroscientists and nutrition experts, we were the go-to family members for advice about what to eat or avoid when taking medications. Even our "family doctor" (Madelyn's brother is a family practice physician) would ask about certain food and medicine interactions for information to give his patients. And doctors with whom we work at the University of Pittsburgh Medical Center told us for years that the basics of what a patient should eat or not eat when taking medications were sorely needed. But, there was no single place to go to for clear and accurate information about the effects of food on medicine. Our colleagues agreed that this would be an important book for us to write, both for consumers and health professionals alike. With Madelyn having broadcast a popular *TODAY Show* segment on this topic, it seemed like a good idea for us to create a one-stop shopping guide for all consumers that lays out the important food and medicine interactions that are known to affect health. Thus, the idea of *Don't Eat This If You're Taking That* was born.

All of us, as patients, often assume that our only job is to take the medicine prescribed to us—to "comply." But while it is essential to take the medication as directed, there are actually many foods that can interfere with the optimal action of a drug—and either boost or block the action. Without even knowing it, we might be getting too much or too little of a medication depending on what foods we choose. That's why this topic is key to supporting good health when we're taking medications. Knowing the importance of this, it may seem surprising that no one has already stepped up to the plate to write a book like this one. However, while it might sound like a simple task to find the information on food and medicine interactions, we found that it is actually quite difficult. There are masses of information in dozens of sources, which are either based on science and medicine, or on opinion and hearsay. Some scientific and medical reports are so complicated that only a medical professional could understand them, while other online sites range from evidence-based, high-quality reports to blends of opinion, half-truths, or just plain wrong information. For most readers, it is often hard to know the difference.

With diligent work, we looked into the facts for the truth about the interactions between certain foods and popular medicines and created this easy-to-understand book. It is for anyone who takes a prescription medication (and some over-the-counter drugs) for a short time, or for years. To make sure you are optimizing the effect of the drug you are taking on your medical condition, you'll want to find the medications you take and learn about what foods and dietary supplements you should avoid or minimize. This book is a must-read if you take a medication yourself, or know someone who does.

To provide the most up-to-date information about food and medicine interactions in a clear and concise way, we have organized the book by the eight most frequently prescribed and used drug categories: antidepressant medicines, pain relief (analgesic) medicines, blood thinner (anticoagulant) medicines, antidiabetes medicines, heartburn (anti-acid reflux) medicines, blood pressure (antihypertensive) medicines, cholesterol-lowering medicines, and heart (cardiovascular) medicines. You'll notice that we've focused on medicines taken orally (no drugs given by injection), since this is where food has the major impact.

This book is especially important for people taking more than one medicine. What you'll find here is an easy format for learning more about the various medications and basic information about what the medicine is actually doing in your body, so you'll be able to translate this information readily into your own life. We've included stories from individuals with multiple health backgrounds to point out the everyday issues that many people have with managing the sometimes surprising impact of foods and dietary supplements on medication effects. Everyone has questions and concerns about food and medicine interactions, and no question is too small to address.

We're thrilled that this information is finally all in one place! No more online searches with vague guidelines and questionable science behind the advice. We are big fans of the "one-stop shopping approach." And when information is presented in a clear and easy-to-understand way, the biological complexities of food and medicine interactions become understandable. We are also strong believers in the idea that when you understand both *how* and *why* a medication works, you'll be more empowered and better able to use your medications to optimize your treatment results. When it comes to eating, we want you to make the best choices not only for healthy eating but also to optimally support, not antagonize, the actions of your medications.

You can be confident that there *are* practical solutions when dietary adjustments need to be made to support optimal efficacy of the medicine. We are all adaptable as human beings—and with food and medicine interactions, it's mostly an issue of finding the right information and knowing how to integrate it into your daily life. We eat every day, and take medicines regularly every day, so, like it or not, it's important to make sure food and medication work together to create optimal health.

Each chapter also includes "Dietary Supplement Alert" boxes that might surprise you. In this book, we count dietary supplements as foods, because they are taken by mouth and typically contain concentrated amounts of one or more nutrients or other bioactive compounds found in foods (vitamin C, for example). We also count herbal extracts from plants, because a law passed by the United States Congress includes them in its definition of "dietary supplement" (The Dietary Supplement Health and Education Act of 1994). While we don't think of them as food items (they aren't), many people include them in their diet, and many have important effects on the prescription drugs we take. We're spending hundreds of millions of dollars on them every year, with more than three-quarters of the population taking at least one dietary supplement. However, the name "supplement" says it all: these products are only meant to supplement, not replace, foods or healthy eating. And, supplements taken in large amounts can have a totally different biological meaning to the body than they do when consumed at normal amounts as components of foods. Sometimes, the "more is better" approach can backfire and lead to negative health consequences.

When it comes to dietary supplements, many people think that these compounds "can't hurt," but the truth is that many contain active ingredients that can affect the same body processes that medications do. And that's the problem—because there is little regulation of dietary supplements (a consequence of the 1994 law identified above), you can't be sure of the purity or the amount of any ingredient present in most products. There might be a useful "active ingredient," but there might also be unknown contaminants produced in the extraction and processing of the supplement that are harmful. Or, the dosage of the "active ingredient" might be much more or less than stated on the package. Simply reading the ingredient list and recommended dosage is not always reliable. And the fact that many of these compounds *do* have biological activity raises a red flag, because using them can affect the function of many medications.

When you're thinking about food and medicine interactions, add dietary supplements to your list of things to limit or avoid. While hundreds of dietary and herbal supplements are available, we've taken the most popular ones and included advice on which to avoid taking with certain commonly used medications. In the alerts section of every chapter we've included the possible effects of combining supplements with medications, focusing on those supplements that are most likely to influence the effects of such medications. For vitamins and minerals, for example, you'll find information on calcium, magnesium and vitamins C, D and E. For herbal products, you'll find information on the most popular herbal supplements, based on sales: garlic, echinacea, saw palmetto, ginkgo biloba, cranberry, soy, ginseng, black cohosh, St. John's wort, milk thistle, and others. Evidence exists showing that many of these can influence the actions of the most-often prescribed drugs. Taking one or more of these (or others), perhaps for one or more years, can be a game-changer when you're taking prescription medicines. While many of these herbal compounds can positively affect your health when consumed as the original food (such as garlic and ginger), when processed into pills and capsules it's a totally different and potentially risky ball game. In this form and advertised as "concentrated," the amounts can be far greater than anything found in nature. Some of these compounds have definite biological actions and in doses that are 10, 50, or 100 times more than the body would see in food, they can have an effect resembling that of a medicine, not a food.

It is our hope that you use this book as a resource in discussions with your doctor, and that it helps you to begin a continuing dialogue on the importance of the possible interactions between medicines and food and dietary supplements. If you are prescribed a medication with food restrictions because of interactions, you need to speak up if you feel the restrictions are too hard to comply with or you feel it really doesn't matter. An open conversation with your doctor can help determine if there are alternate drugs that might be equally effective, but without the food restrictions. Work with your doctor to make sure you're able to comply with the necessary eating changes for successful medical treatment. Sometimes there is no wiggle room, and the food changes are absolute, but often alternatives are available that might make your lifestyle easier. And when you do need to make dietary adjustments, you'll have *Don't Eat This If You're Taking That* as a step-by-step resource to help you make those adjustments.

# Chapter 1
# ANTIDEPRESSANTS

While antidepressant medicines are well-known options for millions of people, it wasn't too long ago that the symptoms of depression were thought to be "all in your head"—and just a matter of willing yourself to feel better. Whether called "the blues" or melancholia, in the old days, the response to people reaching out for help was "life is tough, learn to cope." But science has shown that nothing could be further from the truth. The treatment of depression and anxiety has been documented for decades to be a combination of biology and behavior that *can* be helped by medicine.

The role of the brain in controlling mood is connected to actual abnormalities in brain chemistry. Small changes in brain chemistry in one or more neurotransmitters (brain chemicals) can produce large changes in mood. For many people, depression is a medical illness that benefits from medical treatment and the use of medicines, along with psychological treatment to help make necessary behavioral changes. It's that one-two punch of treatment that studies show is very effective in treating depression.

Beginning in the 1950s, the first generation of antidepressants—tricyclic antidepressants (TCAs) and monoamine oxidase inhibitors (MAOIs)—was discovered and quickly entered the marketplace. More than 50 years later, these medications are still used to treat certain types of depression. As interest in the connection between brain chemistry and depression continued to develop, a new class of antidepressants was introduced, the result of years of scientific research.

New to the market nearly 30 years after the first medications were introduced, these drugs were named serotonin-selective reuptake inhibitors (SSRIs), to resemble the action they had on brain chemistry. They became widely used because they worked well and had fewer side effects when compared with the earlier medicines. SSRIs are used primarily to treat major depression, but many are very useful for the long-term treatment of anxiety disorders and panic disorders. All are presently in clinical use.

Even more medications have been developed for the treatment of depression. A variation of the SSRIs (which only act on serotonin nerve cells), serotonin-norepinephrine reuptake inhibitors (SNRIs) is a group of drugs that act on two brain chemicals: serotonin and norepinephrine. This next generation of medicines has been shown to be a useful addition to antidepressant treatment options.

Still other antidepressants have been identified that don't fit neatly into one of the broad drug categories above. This is because their action on the brain is somewhat mixed, or not well understood, but they have proven to be good treatment options for some patients.

Everyone's brain is different, so it is a modern medical miracle to have so many drug options to help treat depression. The long-term treatment can be challenging, but the right combination of medication and talk therapy has provided relief for millions of people.

We'll take a look at each of these drug classes separately because of the important differences in how foods and supplements affect their actions.

## MEDICATIONS USED TO TREAT DEPRESSION

Tricyclic antidepressants:
- Amitriptyline (Elavil®)
- Clomipramine (Anafranil®)
- Desipramine (Norpramin®)
- Doxepin (Sinequan®)
- Imipramine (Tofranil®)
- Nortriptyline (Pamelor®)
- Protriptyline (Vivactil®)
- Trimipramine (Surmontil®)

Monoamine oxidase inhibitors:
- Phenelzine (Nardil®)
- Isocarboxazid (Marplan®)
- Tranylcypromine (Parnate®)
- Selegiline (Emsam® [skin patch])

Serotonin-selective reuptake inhibitors:
- Citalopram (Celexa®)
- Escitalopram (Lexapro®)
- Fluoxetine (Prozac®, Sarafem®)
- Fluvoxamine (Luvox®)
- Paroxetine (Paxil®, Paxil CR®, Brisdelle®, Pexeva®)
- Sertraline (Zoloft®)
- Vilazodone (Viibryd®)

Serotonin-Norepinephrine Reuptake Inhibitors
- Duloxetine (Cymbalta®)
- Milnacipran (Savella®)
- Venlafaxine (Effexor®, Effexor XR®)
- Desvenlafaxine (Pristiq®, Khedezla®)

Other Antidepressants
- Bupropion (Aplenzin®, Buproban®, Forfivo XL®, Wellbutrin®, Wellbutrin SR® and XL®, Zyban®)
- Mirtazapine (Remeron®)
- Nefazodone (Serzone®)
- Trazodone (Desyrel®, Oleptro®)

# FOODS TO AVOID WHEN TAKING TRICYCLIC ANTIDEPRESSANTS

Alcohol
Grapefruit
Grapefruit Juice

## *Tricyclic Antidepressants*

Eight different tricyclic antidepressants are available in the United States: amitriptyline (Elavil), clomipramine (Anafranil), desipramine (Norpramin), doxepin (Sinequan), imipramine (Tofranil), nortriptyline (Pamelor), protriptyline (Vivactil), and trimipramine (Surmontil). While in the same medication class, very small differences in their chemical makeup have different effects. That's a great thing when it comes to antidepressants, because individual responses to medication can vary widely. What is a miracle drug for one depressed person might not work for another.

If you begin taking one of these drugs, the daily dose will usually be divided into smaller doses taken throughout the day. After several weeks, once you and your physician have determined whether the medication is working, your doctor may suggest that you take the entire daily dose at one time. The general recommendation is usually shortly before bedtime, because these drugs can make you sleepy soon after you take them.

## Foods to Avoid

Alcohol use can interfere with the delicate balance of choosing a dose of an antidepressant to optimize beneficial effects while minimizing side effects. For example, one of the most common side effects of these medications—drowsiness and dizziness—can be enhanced by alcohol. If you are a heavy drinker, alcohol can affect how the body breaks down these drugs, sometimes causing drug levels to be too high in the body and sometimes too low. Heavy alcohol use can make it quite difficult to determine the proper dose for maximizing beneficial effects, while also minimizing side effects. If you take a tricyclic antidepressant, it is wise to avoid alcohol altogether. Check with your doctor for guidance if you are a heavy alcohol user.

Limit the use of grapefruit and grapefruit juice. Grapefruit blocks the body's ability to break down tricyclic antidepressants, resulting in your body "seeing" too much of the medication—essentially, a higher dose. So, limit your intake of grapefruit products to a single serving each day, such as one-half grapefruit or a small glass of grapefruit juice (6–8 ounces), if you are a grapefruit lover. You can also choose to avoid it altogether. If you don't already consume grapefruit products and take a tricyclic antidepressant, check with your doctor *before* adding any grapefruit products to your diet.

## Dietary Supplements to Avoid

When it comes to dietary supplements, the list of compounds to avoid is long. That's because many of these supplements act on the brain, and antidepressants have multiple actions at different brain sites.

Kava and valerian can increase the drowsiness and sleepiness that occurs when taking these medicines. Kava can also interfere with your liver's ability to break down many of these antidepressants, increasing their concentration in the body, and thus potentially increasing side effects. Kava use should be avoided while you are taking a tricyclic antidepressant. If you already use kava or valerian, and a tricyclic antidepressant is recommended for you by your doctor, be sure to discuss your current use of these supplements with him.

St. John's wort increases the breakdown of several tricyclic antidepressants, reducing their levels in the body and potentially reducing their ability to treat your depression. It's as if your body is seeing a lower dose than intended. If you currently use or are thinking about using St. John's wort and are already taking a tricyclic antidepressant, you should discuss this plan with your physician.

Herbal supplements containing bitter orange or ma huang (ephedra) extracts may increase the risk of high blood pressure and abnormal heartbeat when taken with a tricyclic antidepressant. Ma huang contains ephedrine, while bitter orange contains synephrine—both of which increase blood pressure by stimulating the action of a compound, norepinephrine, on the heart and blood vessels. This occurs because the antidepressant itself stimulates norepinephrine action, which may be increased in the presence of ma huang or bitter orange.

## DIETARY SUPPLEMENT ALERT!

**Avoid When Taking Tricyclic Antidepressants:**

Kava
Valerian
St. John's wort
Bitter orange
Ma huang (ephedra)
Tryptophan
5-hydroxytryptophan

Ma huang is no longer permitted to be sold in the United States because it has been linked to a number of deaths related to abnormal heart function and stroke. But ma huang is readily available online—sourced from different countries, or with undocumented claims that the version being sold is not the same plant as that which was removed from the market. Avoid all sources of ma huang if you are taking a tricyclic antidepressant.

Bitter orange extracts are found in many products and are often used in place of ma huang, since the two herbal supplements have similar actions in the body. The use of bitter orange has not yet been linked to the same effects on the heart as ma huang, but has been shown to have an effect on the heart. Its effects may be greater if you are taking a tricyclic antidepressant, so the use of products containing bitter orange should be avoided.

Tryptophan and 5-hydroxytryptophan supplements should be avoided because they raise serotonin levels in the body. This effect will enhance one of the same actions of several of the tricyclic antidepressants, which is to increase the action of serotonin in the brain and elsewhere. It is very important never to mix medications and supplements that each raise serotonin in the body. This excess of serotonin can trigger the "serotonin syndrome," which is potentially life threatening. Common symptoms include confusion, restlessness, spontaneous muscle contractions, tremor, shivering, and excessive sweating. Always discuss your use of these supplements with your doctor when a tricyclic antidepressant is under consideration as a treatment.

If you take a tricyclic antidepressant, or your doctor is considering prescribing one for you, be sure to discuss with him or her relevant dietary issues (like alcohol or grapefruit) and your current use of dietary and herbal supplements, especially ma huang, bitter orange, St. John's wort, kava, valerian, and certain amino acid supplements (tryptophan, 5-hydroxytryptophan).

## *Monoamine Oxidase Inhibitors*

The monoamine oxidase inhibitors (MAOIs) currently in use in the United States for the treatment of depression are phenelzine (Nardil), isocarboxazid (Marplan) and tranylcypromine (Parnate), which are all taken orally. Another MAOI is selegiline (Emsam), which is administered through a skin patch.

Remember to make a full evaluation of your daily diet and herbal and nutrient supplement use if you are going to take an MAOI. MAOIs have many food and supplement interactions that can produce potentially dangerous effects. *All of these drugs can be taken with or without food, but use the guidelines below to help you identify the specific foods that are important to avoid.*

### Foods to Avoid

**Fermented foods:** *Do not consume fermented foods.* While the term "fermented" might not be familiar, the foods in this group certainly are. These are foods that are purposefully or accidentally allowed to be partially digested by microorganisms. These might sound unsafe to consume under any circumstance, but a fungus (like yeast) or bacterium (like lactobacillus) is undoubtedly involved in the creation of some of the foods you love to eat or drink. The most familiar examples are beer and wine, where yeast is used to create the alcohol in them. Many other foods and condiments gain their distinctive flavors through fermentation, including many flavorful cheeses, aged and cured meats, and soy sauce. For a list of the commonly consumed fermented foods, please see the box on page 14.

These "healthy" microorganisms in food have several natural biological actions. They cause fermentation, turning sugars into alcohol products (like wine and

11

beer) or acid foods (like sour cream and yogurt), but they also break down food proteins and convert some of the amino acids that are released in the process into biologically active chemicals called "biogenic amines." When fermented foods are consumed and digested, and their constituents enter the bloodstream, some of these biogenic amines cause blood pressure to rise. Normally, your body (especially your digestive tract, lungs, and liver) contains large amounts of an enzyme, monoamine oxidase, that rapidly destroys these amines, making these foods safe to eat. But if you take a monoamine oxidase inhibitor, this defense mechanism has been turned off, and these biogenic amines are free to enter the body and ultimately produce potentially dangerous effects.

**Alcohol, caffeine, and natural licorice:** Limit your intake of these items to minimize potential side effects of the MAOIs. Alcohol can enhance the sleepiness and loss of concentration that these drugs can cause as a side effect. Limit your daily intake of all caffeine-containing beverages to moderate amounts— no more than 300 milligrams (mg) per day, about two cups of brewed coffee. Excessive intake of caffeine can boost the blood pressure-raising side effect occasionally seen with this group of drugs. And if you eat natural licorice regularly, even in moderate amounts, cut back on your intake. Natural licorice raises blood pressure by causing salt and water retention in the body. When taking a monoamine oxidase inhibitor, you always want to avoid any foods or supplements that have the potential to raise your blood pressure.

━━ Do *not* consume fermented food products and improperly stored food items that can spoil if you take a monoamine oxidase inhibitor. Your doctor should give you careful instructions on how to safely manage this issue. A visit with a registered dietician might also be recommended. And limit or avoid products containing alcohol, caffeine, or licorice.

## FOODS TO AVOID WHEN TAKING MONOAMINE OXIDASE INHIBITORS

- Air-dried, aged, or fermented meats
- Dried sausage and salami
- Liver (especially chicken liver)
- Pickled herring, anchovies, caviar, and shrimp paste
- Soy beans, soy sauce, tofu, miso soup, and bean curd
- Fava beans or pods
- Sauerkraut
- Yeast extracts (including Marmite®, Vegemite®, brewer's yeast, nutritional yeast)
- Meat tenderizers and protein extracts
- Red wine, champagne, beer (from a tap), unpasteurized beer
- Sour cream and strong, aged, or processed cheeses (including blue, brie, cheddar, parmesan, Romano, and Swiss)
- Any spoiled, improperly stored, or "leftover" beef, poultry, fish, or liver
- Figs, raisins, bananas, avocados, and papaya products.
- Chocolate
- *Limit* natural licorice, alcohol, and caffeine

**Dietary supplements:** *Do not take dietary supplements containing the amino acids phenylalanine, tyrosine, dopa, tryptophan or 5-hydroxytryptophan.* Tryptophan, phenylalanine, and tyrosine are converted to transmitter molecules in neurons that normally use them. Dopa and 5-hydroxytryptophan are converted to transmitter molecules as well, but show up in parts of the body that normally do not see them. When they do, they are quickly eliminated by monoamine oxidase. All of these amino acids can also be converted to small amounts of other biogenic amines that the body normally eliminates very quickly, because they produce adverse effects (such as raising blood pressure). The biogenic amines produced from phenylalanine and tyrosine are phenylethylamine, tyramine, and octopamine, while the one produced from tryptophan is tryptamine.

The enzyme responsible for quickly clearing these biogenic amines is monoamine oxidase. While you are taking a monoamine oxidase inhibitor, this defense mechanism is turned off, and when these amino acid supplements are turned into these amines, your body cannot destroy them. Their levels build up in your blood and in some tissues, raise blood pressure, and produce many other undesirable effects. If you take one or more of these amino acids, you should discuss this practice with your doctor before contemplating taking a monoamine oxidase inhibitor. If you are already taking a monoamine oxidase inhibitor, don't start taking any of these amino acids without first talking to your doctor.

**Herbal supplements:** *Do not take herbal supplements containing ma huang or bitter orange.* Ma huang and bitter orange naturally contain biogenic amines that raise blood pressure. Ma huang contains ephedrine, while bitter orange contains synephrine and octopamine. These biogenic amines can raise blood pressure and produce other undesirable effects.

---

### DIETARY SUPPLEMENT ALERT!

**Avoid When Taking MAOIs:**

Amino acids (phenylalanine, tyrosine, dopa, tryptophan, 5-hydroxytryptophan)
Ma huang
Bitter orange
St. John's wort

---

Although ma huang is no longer permitted to be sold as a dietary supplement in the United States, it is still available for purchase online, in multiple forms. Bitter orange is available in several forms as a supplement, and its current use has not yet been linked to adverse effects. But the compounds present in bitter orange have the same actions as ma huang. Monoamine oxidase destroys the bioactive amines present in ma huang and bitter orange when they enter the body. But, if you are taking a monoamine oxidase inhibitor, your body is unable to eliminate them, and they can build up and cause dangerous effects. If you use herbal products containing ma huang or bitter orange, it is very important that you tell your physician, and stop using them while taking a monoamine oxidase inhibitor.

**St. John's wort:** *Do not take St John's wort, tryptophan, or 5-hydroxytryptophan.* Never combine supplements that raise serotonin in the body along with medications that act the same way. MAOIs raise serotonin levels in the brain, which contributes to improvement in your mood. If you combine MAOIs with these supplements, you may develop "serotonin syndrome," a life-threatening condition. Symptoms include confusion, restlessness, spontaneous muscle contractions, tremor, shivering, and excessive sweating. If you are taking an MAOI, you need to be especially careful to avoid these compounds, which are all sold as herbal and dietary supplements.

There are a number of herbal supplements and dietary supplements (amino acids) that are available in health food stores and online that usually do not cause harmful effects when ingested. But they can cause great harm to your body if you use them while you are taking a monoamine oxidase inhibitor. Be very vigilant in identifying these compounds in products you may use (read labels), and avoid their use while taking a monoamine oxidase inhibitor. If you have any concerns whatsoever relating to this issue, talk with your doctor.

## *Serotonin-Selective Reuptake Inhibitors*

Sometimes called second generation antidepressants, serotonin-selective reuptake inhibitors (SSRIs) are defined by how they act in the brain: they are more selective in their chemical action on the brain than are the tricyclic antidepressants discussed above, resulting in far fewer side effects, while still being very effective in treating depression. There are two groups of drugs in this newer category of antidepressants. The first group is discussed in this section and has a selective action only on serotonin function in the brain. A second group, SNRIs, acts on both serotonin and norepinephrine activity in the brain and will be discussed later.

The SSRIs in use in the United States are citalopram (Celexa), escitalopram (Lexapro), fluoxetine (Prozac, Sarafem), fluvoxamine (Luvox), paroxetine (Paxil, Paxil CR®, Brisdelle, Pexeva), sertraline (Zoloft), and vilazodone (Viibryd).

While all of the SSRIs are similar in action, they differ somewhat in the kinds of foods and supplements that should be limited or avoided, and how they are taken in relation to food. Citalopram, escitalopram, fluoxetine, fluvoxamine, and paroxetine can all be taken *with or without food.* Vilazodone should be taken *with food*, as food improves its absorption considerably. Sertraline absorption is only modestly increased when ingested with food, so it can be taken with or without food—but you should be consistent one way or the other.

### Foods to Avoid

For starters, there are certain foods to avoid when taking *any* SSRI. *Alcohol* can enhance the common SSRI side effects of drowsiness and dizziness, so limit or avoid alcohol. *Avoid foods that reduce platelet function:* Serotonin plays a key role in platelet function, and SSRIs can reduce platelet function by lowering their content of serotonin. Large amounts of *garlic* and *onion* can also inhibit platelet function, and increase the likelihood of greater bleeding following a cut or contusion. If you are a heavy consumer of either of these foods, reducing your intake of them while taking an SSRI may reduce the likelihood of bleeding.

Some food limitations apply to only some of the drugs in this class. Limit the use of grapefruit and grapefruit juice if you take sertraline or vilazodone, because compounds present in grapefruit inhibit the body's ability to metabolize sertraline and vilazodone. This is a problem only if you ingest large amounts of grapefruit and grapefruit juice. Ingesting large amounts of this fruit or juice each day can increase the amount of drug in your body, which increases the likelihood of negative side effects. If you're a grapefruit lover, the best strategy is to *limit* your intake of these foods to a single serving each day. A single serving means one-half grapefruit or 6–8 ounces of grapefruit juice.

Reduce your intake of caffeine if you take fluvoxamine, the only SSRI that interferes with the breakdown of caffeine in your body. If you take this drug and drink caffeine-containing foods and drinks, caffeine levels in your body may rise beyond normal levels. If you are taking fluvoxamine and notice you are having heightened caffeine effects—such as nervousness, restlessness, stomach upset, increased heart rate, and difficulty sleeping—you should reduce your daily intake of caffeine-containing products.

**Dietary Supplements to Avoid**

**St. John's wort, tryptophan, and 5-hydroxytryptophan**: Because all three of these supplements raise serotonin function in the body, using them while taking an SSRI can lead to the "serotonin syndrome" (symptoms include confusion, restlessness, spontaneous muscle contractions, tremor, shivering, and excessive sweating). Do *not* take *any* of these compounds if you are taking an SSRI. And be sure to discuss this issue with your doctor if he suggests an SSRI medication for the treatment of your depression and you are presently using one or more of these supplements.

---

### DIETARY SUPPLEMENT ALERT!

**Avoid When Using SSRIs:**

St. John's wort
Tryptophan
5-hydroxytryptophan
Vitamin E
Omega-3 fatty acids and fish oil
Ginkgo biloba
Asian ginseng
Bilberry
Ginger
Horse chestnut
Garlic

---

St. John's wort also *decreases* the action of certain SSRIs (citalopram, escitalopram, sertraline, vilazodone) by speeding up their elimination from the body. As a result, blood levels decline, reducing the SSRIs' ability to treat depression successfully. If you take St. John's wort and are prescribed one of these SSRIs, you should stop using this herbal product and inform your physician so that your SSRI dose can be adjusted.

**Vitamins and herbal supplements that inhibit platelet function**: The SSRIs boost mood by elevating serotonin in the brain. But serotonin is also used in other parts of the body to accomplish completely different functions. Platelets contain serotonin, and use it to help initiate clot formation. SSRIs lower the serotonin content in platelets. Without enough serotonin in the platelets, you may find that scrapes and cuts bleed longer than expected. You may also notice that bruising occurs more easily. If you do notice any of these effects, you should talk to your doctor to see if your medication dose needs to be reduced. But you can be proactive and reduce the likelihood of this side effect by reducing the ingestion of supplements that may contribute to the problem. Several supplements can reduce platelet function, including garlic as a supplement, vitamin E in high amounts, and omega-3 fatty acid supplements and fish oil. If you ingest any of these, consider cutting back. You can easily meet your dietary requirement for vitamin E in food each day, so if you take a vitamin E supplement, you should think about stopping. Omega-3 fatty acids are often taken as a fish oil supplement. If you take a fish oil supplement, consider discontinuing it and eating fish two or more times a week instead. Some herbal supplements also are known to inhibit platelet function: ginkgo biloba, Asian ginseng, bilberry, ginger, and horse chestnut. If you use any of these supplements, consider discontinuing their use while you are taking an SSRI.

If you'd like to learn more about foods and supplements that affect platelet function, look on pages 65–79 in chapter 3 for information about blood thinners. And always discuss the appropriate use of all of these dietary supplements and products with your physician, if you are using one or more of them and taking an SSRI.

## *Serotonin-Norepinephrine Reuptake Inhibitors*

Following the successful development and application of SSRI medications (which specifically act on brain serotonin cells) for the treatment of depression, subsequent research identified additional drugs that proved useful in treating depression, the serotonin-norepinephrine reuptake inhibitors (SNRIs). The SNRIs in use in the United States are duloxetine (Cymbalta), milnacipran (Savella), venlafaxine (Effexor, Effexor XR) and desvenlafaxine (Pristiq, Khedezla). They can be taken with or without food.

The same guidelines discussed above for the SSRIs also apply to SNRIs, namely discontinuing the use of alcohol; avoiding St. John's wort, tryptophan, and 5-hydroxytryptophan; and avoiding foods and supplements that inhibit platelet function. They apply because SNRIs affect serotonin in the same way that SSRIs do. Read the SSRI section above for a complete description of foods and supplements to avoid if you are taking an SNRI.

Because these drugs *also* act as norepinephrine reuptake inhibitors, there's more than serotonin to worry about; the interactions with the brain chemical norepinephrine must be addressed. Norepinephrine action as an antidepressant might sound familiar, if you looked at the tricyclic antidepressants section. The SNRIs and the tricyclic drugs have a common effect— to boost the action of norepinephrine—so the same concerns about norepinephrine interactions apply to their use.

As discussed above in greater detail, ma huang contains ephedrine, and bitter orange contains synephrine and octopamine. The use of either with an SNRI drug could boost norepinephrine action enough to raise blood pressure and cause an abnormal heartbeat. *If you take one of the SNRIs, avoid supplements that contain ma huang or bitter orange.*

## *Other Antidepressants*

The following widely used antidepressants do not fit neatly into one of the function-oriented categories already discussed: bupropion (Aplenzin, Buproban, Forfivo XL, Wellbutrin, Wellbutrin SR and XL, Zyban), mirtazapine (Remeron), nefazodone (Serzone) and trazodone (Desyrel, Oleptro). They all have different actions to improve depression, so we discuss them separately to avoid confusion. Many are related to the SSRI and SNRI drugs, so we refer back to other sections in this chapter as needed for a more detailed explanation.

Bupropion (Aplenzin, Buproban, Forfivo XL, Wellbutrin, Wellbutrin SR and XL, Zyban) is a norepinephrine-dopamine reuptake inhibitor. It can be taken with or without food. You should not take this drug if you are a heavy user of alcoholic beverages, because stopping alcohol use abruptly while taking this drug can lead to an increased chance of seizures. Discuss your use of alcohol with your doctor regarding this drug or any antidepressant.

Mirtazapine (Remeron) has multiple chemical actions, but important among them is the stimulation of serotonin and norepinephrine function in the brain (like the SSRIs and SNRIs). For this reason, the dietary and supplement precautions are the same as for SSRIs and SNRIs. Read those sections above for more details. Briefly, if you take mirtazapine, avoid alcohol, kava and valerian, as they will make you drowsier. Since mirtazapine increases serotonin function, you should avoid taking St. John's wort, tryptophan, and 5-hydroxytryptophan with this drug. The combination of mirtazapine with one or more of these supplements may cause the "serotonin syndrome," described in earlier sections, which is potentially life threatening.

Nefazodone (Serzone) also has several chemical actions, *one* of which is as an SSRI. The same concerns about the SSRI drugs thus apply generally to this drug. Nefazodone can be taken with or without food, although taking it with food is known to reduce the side effect of light-headedness some people experience when taking it on an empty stomach. Alcohol should also not be consumed with this drug, as it can increase the drowsiness sometimes produced by the drug itself. Because nefazodone increases serotonin function, avoid using St. John's wort, tryptophan, and 5-hydroxytryptophan while taking this drug, as any combination can increase the risk of developing the potentially dangerous "serotonin syndrome."

Trazodone (Desyrel, Oleptro) is similar in structure to nefazodone, with multiple actions, including as an SSRI. It can be taken with or without food, but taking it with food will reduce the occurrence of stomach upset and light-headedness. If you take trazodone, avoid alcohol, and also St. John's wort, tryptophan, and 5-hydroxytryptophan. In addition, if you consume grapefruit or grapefruit juice in large amounts, you should reduce your intake to one serving a day (one-half grapefruit *or* a 6–8-ounce glass of grapefruit juice). The consumption of large amounts of grapefruit or grapefruit juice slows the metabolism of trazodone in the body, which can increase the occurrence of side effects. Avoid using ginkgo biloba, as its use has been reported to cause drowsiness in subjects taking trazodone.

## PATIENT STORY: ROBERT

Robert's wife had died after a long illness, and he was now a single dad with two teenage sons, in addition to his career as an accountant. While he expected a long period of grief, he counted on family and friends to help him transition to the "new normal." While Robert wasn't sure how long it would take, he figured he would manage all right and focused on his family and his work. But after 10 months, he still had a great deal of trouble sleeping and concentrating, and often found it hard to get through the day. He felt exhausted, and the boys were getting *him* up in the morning. Robert thought he needed some help but was embarrassed to talk to his doctor about it. He figured he should be able to tough it out.

His friend suggested St. John's wort, which was described to him as a type of vitamin to help depressive symptoms. Robert took that dietary supplement daily for six weeks, but his symptoms did not improve. He told his sister, Sally, about it, and she insisted he see his doctor—and accompanied him for moral support.

Robert discussed his symptoms, and his doctor diagnosed him with mild depression. He prescribed a trial of the SSRI paroxetine (Paxil). His doctor told him to start the Paxil—but not until two weeks after stopping the St. John's wort because this supplement could boost the action of the Paxil and cause unwanted side effects.

His Paxil trial was a success. After about 14 days, he noticed he had more good days than bad ones, and that he seemed to have more energy. Robert went back to running two–three miles a day. His sons were thrilled; they were a family again—dad was back.

His sister also suggested he support the medication with talk therapy, an idea Robert had never been keen on. He did hear about a bereavement group, which interested him because he liked the option of just listening. The group was a good support outlet for him and, along with the medication, helped him through his depression. Now six months into treatment, Robert reports feeling more like himself. He plans to talk with his doctor soon to determine whether it's a good idea to stay on the medication or perhaps lowering the dosage, eventually tapering off. Robert and his doctor agree that for now, paroxetine is a health-promoting tool for him.

## PATIENT STORY: ELLEN

Ellen had a history of depression since her college years and, at age 35, still couldn't find the right combination of treatments. She was a big fan of talk therapy, which had been helping her for years. But therapy alone was not enough. She had tried several SSRIs that helped, but they also had the negative side effect of causing unwanted weight gain. She was determined not to have this happen again—she had spent two years losing those extra 30 pounds.

She was off and on medication but maintained therapy for years. She told her current psychiatrist she really did not want to take another medicine that might cause weight gain as a side effect. Ellen was doing well in therapy and agreed with her doctor that a trial of bupropion was a good idea to support talk therapy. This medication is generally well tolerated, and not associated with weight gain. Ellen began Wellbutrin XL, and in about two weeks reported feeling somewhat better. She also liked the fact that she didn't have that weird "out of body" mental experience she had with SSRIs; she felt very connected to the world. Ellen has continued on Wellbutrin XL for more than a year, and with weekly group therapy, she is feeling well.

# Chapter 2
# PAIN RELIEF (Analgesic) MEDICINES

None of us wants to hear the word "pain" without the word "relief" attached to it. While we all say we feel pain and seek medications to relieve pain and discomfort, that's not exactly what's happening in our bodies. What this group of drugs actually does is reduce our perception of pain. Does this mean that pain isn't real? Not at all! To understand how pain medications, called "analgesics," work, it's important to learn more about how the body recognizes and responds to pain.

Pain can occur when body parts are damaged either on the outside (external) or on the inside (internal). Think of a knife cut on your finger, falling and scraping your knee, or the crush resulting from dropping a heavy object on your foot. These are all external sources of pain. If you have an infection (like herpes zoster, the virus that causes shingles), cancer, broken bones, or joint pain, just to name a few, you'll also experience intense and often chronic pain. These are all internal sources of pain, originating inside the body.

In both cases, the perception of pain occurs *in* the brain, although the painful event has occurred *outside* of the brain. For the brain to perceive pain, it first receives a signal from the injured part of the body. This occurs when a special type of nerve cell senses damage. These sensing cells (sensory neurons) are all over the body and have long, wire-like parts that send pain signals from the injury site into your spinal cord, then up into the brain. These connections can be very long, reaching from your toes into your spinal cord. Your spinal cord and brain cells receive these signals and together act like a computer to analyze them and create the feeling of pain that you perceive—which alerts you to the problem. Once you become aware of the problem, you can identify the source and site of the pain, and attend to the damage.

But why should the body have a pain-generating system? We'd be better off without it, you might say. No pain would be a good thing, right? Wrong. Whether the pain is from a burn, a broken bone, back pain, diabetic nerve pain, or many other causes, feeling the sensation of pain and responding to it protects us from injury and body damage. If we could not perceive pain, we could not respond to dangerous situations and protect ourselves from harm (think of placing your hand on a very hot stove). And if we did not feel anything from an injury and left it unattended, parts of the body could become permanently damaged.

However, when these pain-sensing systems go into overdrive, and the pain is so intense that it interferes with daily living, pain medications are often part of the solution. The perception of pain and the ability to tolerate it is highly variable from person to person. A wealth of scientific literature indicates that both biology and individual behavior contribute to each individual's tolerance to pain and his or her response to pain medications. That's why pain management is so challenging, with medical specialists devoted to developing optimal strategies to help people manage both short-term and chronic pain.

Analgesic drugs reduce the perception of pain by *turning down* the responsiveness of nerve cells that sense pain throughout the body and alert the brain. With a weaker signal, the brain generates a less intense pain alarm that reaches your consciousness, and thus you experience less discomfort. There are four major classes of analgesic drugs that accomplish this effect, each acting through different chemical mechanisms. These drugs are available as over-the-counter nonprescription medications and, in some cases, by prescription only. (Some of the drugs that are nonprescription become prescription-only medications when available at higher doses.)

The most widely used analgesic drug classes right now are nonsteroidal anti-inflammatory drugs (NSAIDs), opioids (also called "opiates"), drugs for treating migraine headache attacks, and drugs for treating neuropathic pain (like diabetic neuropathy and herpes).

To make it easier for you to find your own medication—this is a big category—we've listed all of the specific medications in each of these four categories in the boxes on pages 34–36 according to how they act in the body to relieve pain. Once you've found your drug and its "group," look for this group term in the chapter for the kinds of foods and dietary supplements you need to pay attention to. We're using the specific drug name in the box, so you can readily find your personal category—making it a lot easier for you to find potential interactions.

## FOUR CATEGORIES OF PAIN RELIEF MEDICATIONS

Nonsteroidal anti-inflammatory drugs:
- Acetaminophen
  Tylenol®
  Cetafen®
- Salicylates
  Acetylsalicylic acid (Aspirin [all
      brands])
  Magnesium salicylate (Doan's pills®)
  Difunisal (Dolobid®)
  Salsalate (Disalcid®)
- Nonselective cyclooxygenase
      inhibitors
  Diclofenac (Cambia®, Cataflam®,
      Voltaren XR®, Zipsor®, Zorvolex®)
  Etodolac (Lodine®, Lodine® XL)
  Fenoprofen (Nalfon®)
  Flurbiprofen (Ansaid®)
  Ibuprofen (Advil®, Motrin®)
  Indomethacin (Indocin®)
  Ketoprofen (Orovail®, Orudis®)
  Ketorolac (Toradol®)
  Meclofenamate (Meclomen®)
  Mefenamic acid (Ponstel®)
  Meloxicam (Mobic®)
  Nabumetone (Relafen®)
  Naproxen (Aleve®, Naprosyn®,
      Anaprox®, Naprelan®)
  Oxaprozin (Daypro®)

Piroxicam (Feldene®)
Sulindac (Clinoril®)
Tolmetin (Tolectin®)
• Selective cyclooxygenase-2 inhibitors
Celecoxib (Celebrex®)

Opioids (opiates):
Buprenorphine (Buprenex®, Butrans®)
Butalbital (Fiorinal®, Fioricet® [combined
with aspirin and caffeine])
Butorphanol (Stadol®)
Codeine
Fentanyl (Fentora®, Actiq®, Onsolis®,
Abstral®, Lazanda®)
Hydrocodone (Hysingla ER®,
Zohydro ER®; Vicodin® [with
acetaminophen]; Hydrocodone with
ibuprofen [Ibudone®, Reprexain®,
Vicoprofen®])
Hydromorphone (Dilaudid®,
Dilaudid-HP®, Exalgo®)
Levorphanol (Levo-Dromoran®)
Meperidine (Demerol®, Meperitab®)
Methadone (Dolophine®, Methadose®)
Morphine sulfate (Avinza®, Kadian®, MS
Contin®, Roxanol®)
Oxycodone (Oxycontin®, Oxecta®,
Roxicodone®, Percoset®, Roxicet®;
Tylox® [with acetaminophen];
Percodan® [with aspirin])
Oxymorphone (Opana®, Opana ER®)

Tapentadol (Nucynta®, Nucynta ER®)
Tramadol (Ultram®, Ultram ER®,
    ConZip®, Synapryn®; Ultracet® [with
    acetaminophen])

Migraine headache medications:
    Almotriptan (Axert®)
    Eletriptan (Relpax®)
    Frovatriptan (Frova®)
    Naratriptan (Amerge®)
    Rizatriptan (Maxalt®, Maxalt MLT®)
    Sumatriptan (Imitrex®; Treximet®
        [with naproxen])
    Zolmitriptan (Zomig®, Zomig-ZMT®)

Nerve pain medications:
    Pregabalin (Lyrica®)
    Gabapentin (Neurontin®, Gralise®)
    Gabapentin enacarbil (Horizant®)
    Select antidepressants (some TCAs,
        and SNRIs)

## *Nonsteroidal anti-inflammatory drugs*

Nonsteroidal anti-inflammatory drug (NSAID) is a general name for four different types of medication that all act the same way to relieve pain: acetaminophen, salicylates, nonselective cyclooxygenase inhibitors, and selective cyclooxygenase-2 inhibitors. They all block the production of a type of natural chemical found throughout your body that activates pain signals. These chemicals, prostaglandins, have two actions on the brain that stimulate pain, so when they are blocked, the pain is reduced. It's a simple concept, but it took scientists many years of research to discover these chemicals and how they work, and then to develop effective drugs to block the pain signals they generate.

These medications reduce the sensation of pain anywhere in the body because they block both actions of the pain-promoting prostaglandins. It's a one-two punch for pain relief. First, they block the prostaglandin signal that appears at the damaged body part. This signal tickles the sensory neurons that send the brain a signal that there is pain. And second, these medications blunt the brain's perception that a painful signal was delivered—further reducing the strength of any pain signal that you ultimately perceive.

Some of these drugs are available over the counter in the United States at nonprescription strength, including acetaminophen (Tylenol), acetylsalicylic acid (aspirin), magnesium salicylate (Doan's Pills), ibuprofen (Advil, Motrin), and naproxen (Aleve). There are many others available only by prescription.

## Acetaminophen

Acetaminophen is found in many brands, including Acephen, Cetafen, and Tylenol. But be sure to check *all* product labels for acetaminophen as an active ingredient to be certain. This may be taken with or without food. If you use this drug regularly, do not exceed the total daily dose listed on the product, unless your doctor has told you to do so. This is usually around 3,000 mg. (In some formulations, this would be 10 pills per day, each pill containing 325 mg.) And avoid using this product if you consume three or more alcoholic drinks each day. At doses above 4,000 mg daily, acetaminophen can damage your liver. This effect can be worsened by consuming significant amounts of alcohol regularly. While three or more drinks a day is already a health negative, if you do consume this much, choose another pain reliever in this grouping to avoid potential further damage to your liver.

## Salicylates

The drugs in this class are acetylsalicylic acid (aspirin, which is also present in many combination products— check for it as an ingredient in all pain relief products), difunisal (Dolobid), magnesium salicylate (Doan's Pills), and salsalate (Disalcid). Aspirin can be safely taken with or without food. Many people choose to take aspirin along with food, if they experience an upset stomach. Enteric coated aspirin (Ecotrin®) largely eliminates stomach upset, since the tablet does not dissolve and release the aspirin until it passes through the stomach into the intestines.

If you take plain aspirin (not enteric coated) on a regular basis, reduce or eliminate alcohol intake, as alcohol can increase the chance of stomach bleeding in combination with aspirin. Be sure to ask your doctor about using alcohol even in moderation while you are taking aspirin, especially if you regularly take aspirin by prescription.

Salicylates inhibit platelet function and therefore can impede clot formation and increase the risk of bleeding. If you take aspirin more than occasionally, particularly if by prescription, you should avoid or reduce the ingestion of dietary supplements that also inhibit blood platelet function.

A main inhibitor of normal platelet activity and clot formation is vitamin E. High doses are required to produce this action, much higher than is consumed in the normal diet. If you consume a normal diet along with a standard daily multivitamin containing vitamin E, there is no added risk. But if you take a large daily dose of supplemental vitamin E for any other reason, and your doctor prescribes a salicylate to be taken chronically, you should tell him that you take supplemental vitamin E, and the daily dose. Your doctor will determine if you need to moderate your use of vitamin E. (For more on vitamin E requirements, go to chapter 3, page 66.)

Another supplement that should be avoided are the omega-3 fatty acids. Found in some fish and in fish oils (marine oils), they can reduce platelet function and slow the blood clotting mechanism when they are consumed as a supplement, resulting in an increased risk of bleeding. Eating fish as part of a healthy diet is not a concern, but daily fish oil or omega-3 fatty acid-containing supplements taken together with a prescription-strength dose of a salicylate may increase the likelihood of bleeding. Be sure to tell your doctor if you are using these supplements, and how much. You may be asked to reduce your intake of them.

*Onion* and *garlic* contain compounds that interfere with platelet activity and normal blood clotting. Their ingestion in large amounts—in foods or in supplement form—may boost the antiplatelet and anti-blood-clotting actions of salicylates. If your doctor prescribes a prescription strength salicylate for chronic use, and you regularly consume large amounts of onion or garlic, or take these as supplements, speak up! You may be asked to moderate your intake while taking these drugs.

A number of other herbal supplements inhibit platelet function and normal blood clotting. That's why it is important to discuss *all* of the herbal supplements you use with your doctor before beginning salicylate treatment. You may be asked to stop taking the supplements that are linked to excessive bleeding. Herbal supplements thought to inhibit platelet function include Asian ginseng, bilberry, cocoa, danshen, ginger, ginkgo biloba, and horse chestnut. You can look online to identify others at Drugs.com, WebMD (webmd.com), the National Center for Complementary and Integrative Health website (nccih.nih.gov/health/herbsataglance.htm), and the website of the Office of Dietary Supplements, National Institutes of Health (ods.od.nih.gov/factsheets/list-all/).

## Nonselective Cyclooxygenase Inhibitors

Some of the most popular medications in this group include ibuprofen (Advil, Motrin) and naproxen (Aleve, Naprosyn, Anaprox, Naprelan). Other drugs in this class are diclofenac (Cambia, Cataflam, Voltaren XR, Zipsor, Zorvolex), etodolac (Lodine, Lodine XL), fenoprofen (Nalfon), flurbiprofen (Ansaid), indomethacin (Indocin), ketoprofen (Oruvail, Orudis), ketorolac (Toradol), meclofenamate (Meclomen), mefenamic acid (Ponstel), meloxicam (Mobic), nabumetone (Relafen), oxaprozin (Daypro), piroxicam (Feldene), sulindac (Clinoril) and tolmetin (Tolectin).

All of these drugs can be taken on an empty stomach, with a glass of water. But if you experience stomach irritation or upset, taking food with these drugs should minimize the upset. And reducing your caffeine intake can also help reduce stomach irritation with these drugs. Check with your doctor, since the potency of some of these medicines—diclofenac, meclofenamate, and naproxen—may be reduced somewhat if consumed with food.

When you are taking one of these drugs, your doctor may ask you to reduce your alcohol consumption because it can increase the possibility of stomach bleeding while taking them. These medications may also make you dizzy or drowsy. If you find this to be the case, tell your doctor. You may need to change drugs, or eliminate alcohol altogether from your diet.

Like the salicylates, all of the nonselective cyclooxygenase inhibitors inhibit platelet function and reduce the ability of your blood to clot normally, thus increasing the risk of bleeding. While you are taking one of these drugs, you should avoid or greatly limit your intake of dietary supplements that also block platelet function. These are all of the same compounds discussed above for the salicylates, namely *vitamin E* (which is okay if taken as a multivitamin, but not as a high-dose supplement), *fish oil* or *omega-3 fatty acid* supplements (fish is okay), *garlic* and *onion* in large amounts or in the form of a supplement, and a variety of herbal supplements (notably Asian ginseng, bilberry, cocoa, danshen, ginger, ginkgo biloba, and horse chestnut). It is important to discuss this issue with your doctor if you are a regular user of one or more of these supplements and are taking a medicine in this group.

## Selective Cyclooxygenase-2 Inhibitors

Presently, there is only one drug in this category approved for use in the United States, celecoxib (Celebrex). This drug is taken along with a glass of water, but may be taken with milk or food, if you experience stomach irritation or upset. Celebrex *does not inhibit platelet function at normally prescribed doses.* It is still a good idea to discuss your use of vitamin E and herbal supplements with your doctor, in case new information develops. This is the only one of the four groups of NSAIDs that has not been shown to interfere with platelet activity and clotting activity but new information could prove otherwise. It's better to be proactive so your doctor knows all of your daily supplements.

**FOODS TO AVOID WHEN TAKING PAIN RELIEF MEDICATIONS**

With NSAIDS:
- Alcohol
- Onion and garlic (in large amounts or supplement form), with salicylates and nonselective cyclooxygenase inhibitors only

With opioids:
- Alcohol
- Grapefruit and grapefruit juice

## *Opioids*

The opioid (opiate) category of pain relievers is very effective, but they are addictive and their use is carefully regulated by the federal government. When your doctor prescribes an opioid for intense pain, it's essential to follow the dosing instructions carefully.

Opioids act within the spinal cord and brain at sites involved in transmitting a pain signal into a conscious feeling of pain. These medicines reduce the perception of pain signals and how you react to them. There are many drugs in this group, and some are combined with an NSAID for greater pain-relieving action (by providing two different ways that pain is handled by the body): buprenorphine (Buprenex, Butrans); butalbital (Fiorinal; Fioricet [combined with aspirin and caffeine]); butorphanol (Stadol), codeine, fentanyl (Fentora, Actiq, Onsolis, Abstral, Lazanda); hydrocodone (Hysingla ER, Zohydro ER; Vicodin [with acetaminophen]; Ibudone, Reprexain, and Vicoprofen [with ibuprofen]); hydromorphone (Dilaudid, Dilaudid-HP, Exalgo), levorphanol, meperidine (Demerol, Meperitab), methadone (Dolophine, Methadose), morphine sulfate (Avinza, Kadian, MS Contin, Roxanol), oxycodone (Oxycontin, Oxecta, Roxicodone, Percoset, Roxicet; Tylox [with acetaminophen]; Percodan [with aspirin]), oxymorphone (Opana, Opana ER), tapentadol (Nucynta, Nucynta ER), and tramadol (Ultram, Ultram ER, ConZip, Synapryn; Ultracet [with acetaminophen]).

With a few exceptions, the opioids can be taken with or without food. Many people experience stomach upset on an empty stomach, so, for some, it may be more agreeable to take these with food. There are several important exceptions. For oxycodone or oxymorphone, ingestion with a high-fat meal can increase drug absorption and boost the drug effect for the same dose. Check with your doctor if you are prescribed either of these drugs to see if you should avoid taking your pill with meals containing fat. Similarly, the absorption of morphine sulfate in liquid form (Roxanol) is increased if taken with food. If you are prescribed this form of morphine, ask your doctor when to take it in relation to food.

All opioids can make you drowsy, dizzy, and lightheaded. For this reason, you should avoid alcoholic beverages, which can increase this effect. The herbal supplements kava and valerian also cause drowsiness, so stop using them while you are taking an opioid. In addition, do *not* take Avinza, Kadian (extended-release morphine sulfate), Opana ER (extended-release oxymorphone), or Nucynta ER (extended-release tapentadol) with alcohol, as blood levels of the drug can become dangerously elevated when combined with alcohol.

The activity of some opioids can be reduced by the herbal supplement St. John's wort. If you take buprenorphine, codeine, fentanyl, hydrocodone, methadone, oxycodone, or tramadol, you should not use St. John's wort while you are taking the opioid because the drug may not work as well. In contrast, the activity of other opioids can be increased by consuming grapefruit or grapefruit juice. If you are prescribed fentanyl, hydrocodone, methadone or oxycodone, stop eating grapefruit and drinking grapefruit juice while you are on the medication. The effect of the opioid may become greater, and side effects may become more prominent; among the most dangerous is a slowing down of your rate of breathing.

Some opioids are formulated with added acetaminophen, aspirin, or ibuprofen. These drugs have their own set of side effects and dietary interactions, as discussed above for the NSAID group. If your doctor prescribes one of these combination opioids, you need to have an open discussion about the possible side effects at the dose you will be taking, along with potential interactions with food and herbal supplements.

For *acetaminophen*, the opioid formulations are butalbital (Fioricet), hydrocodone (Vicodin), oxycodone (Percoset, Roxicet, Tylox), and tramadol (Ultracet). At high acetaminophen doses (more than 4,000 mg daily), this drug combination can cause liver toxicity. Since alcohol can also enhance the liver toxicity potential of acetaminophen, alcohol should be avoided if you are taking one of the opioid formulations that contains acetaminophen.

For *aspirin*, the opioid formulations are butalbital (Fiorinal) and oxycodone (Percodan). These can cause diminished platelet function (and bleeding), which can be aggravated by vitamin E and omega-3 fatty acids, garlic, and onion in large amounts or in the form of a supplement, and many herbal supplements, including Asian ginseng, bilberry, cocoa, danshen, ginger, ginkgo biloba, and horse chestnut.

For *ibuprofen*, there is one opioid formulation: hydrocodone (Ibudone, Reprexain, Vicoprofen). The concern with ibuprofen is also diminished platelet function, as for the aspirin-containing opioid preparations, and the dietary and herbal supplement issues are thus the same as those listed immediately above.

# DIETARY SUPPLEMENT ALERT!

## Avoid When Taking Pain Relief Medications:

With NSAIDS:
- Vitamin E
- Fish oil (omega-3-fats)
- Onion and garlic supplements
- Asian ginseng
- Bilberry
- Cocoa
- Danshen
- Ginger
- Ginkgo biloba
- Horse chestnut

With opioids:
- Kava
- Valerian
- St. John's wort

With migraine medications:
- St. John's wort
- 5-HTP (5-hydroxytryptophan)

Nerve (neuropathic) pain medications:
- Kava
- Valerian

## Migraine Drugs

For anyone who suffers from migraine headaches, the development of effective prescription drugs to relieve pain is a medical miracle. Over-the-counter analgesics simply do not have the potency to manage the intensity of the pain signals. And combining migraine drugs with some smart lifestyle changes creates a multifaceted approach to optimize migraine headache management.

A migraine headache is currently thought to occur when a particular network of nerve cells in the brain that processes pain signals becomes active on its own— in the absence of an input of pain signals from those cells that "sense" pain in certain parts of the body outside of the brain. While it remains unclear how this particular cascade of pain signals occurs in the brain, it is known that the start of a migraine headache somehow begins within the brain itself. The perceived pain can be quite debilitating and impairs daily living for millions of people. Because of this, the search for drug treatments has been ongoing for more than 100 years, with only partial success.

But now there is some good news: a recently identified group of drugs, the *triptans*, appears to be quite effective for many sufferers. The triptans are almotriptan (Axert), eletriptan (Relpax), frovatriptan (Frova), naratriptan (Amerge), rizatriptan (Maxalt, Maxalt MLT), sumatriptan (Imitrex; Treximet [contains sumatriptan and naproxen]), and zolmitriptan (Zomig, Zomig-ZMT). All of these drugs can be taken with or without food.

## MEDICATIONS USED TO TREAT MIGRAINE HEADACHES

Almotriptan (Axert®)
Eletriptan (Relpax®)
Frovatriptan (Frova®)
Naratriptan (Amerge®)
Rizatriptan (Maxalt®, Maxalt MLT®)
Sumatriptan (Imitrex®)
Sumatriptan Plus Naproxen (Treximet®)
Zolmitriptan (Zomig®, Zomig-ZMT®)
Ergotamine (Ergomar®)
Ergotamine plus caffeine (Cafergot®)
Dihydroergotamine plus caffeine (Migranal®)

Only some of the triptan medications have food restrictions. If you take almotriptan (Axert) or eletriptan (Relpax), you should stop eating grapefruit or drinking grapefruit juice. Grapefruit can cause a significant increase in the blood levels of these drugs, as if your body is "seeing" a higher dose. This can increase the likelihood of negative side effects. If you are a grapefruit lover, discuss this with your doctor, who may change your medication for one in this group that does not have an interaction with grapefruit.

**AVOID GRAPEFRUIT AND
GRAPEFRUIT JUICE WITH THESE
MIGRAINE DRUGS**

Almotriptan (Axert®)
Eletriptan (Relpax®)
Ergotamine (Ergomar®)
Ergotamine plus caffeine (Cafergot®)
Dihydroergotamine plus caffeine (Migranal®)

Triptans also interact with two popular dietary supplements: St. John's wort and 5-hydroxytryptophan. If you take either of these supplements, you should discontinue using them while taking any of the triptans. The combination can cause an excess of serotonin activity in the brain, which is potentially very dangerous as it can lead to the "serotonin syndrome." Common symptoms include confusion, restlessness, spontaneous muscle contractions, tremor, shivering, and excessive sweating.

---

### DIETARY SUPPLEMENTS ALERT!

**Avoid When Taking Migraine Medications:**

St. John's wort
5-hydroxytryptophan

---

While the newer triptan family of medications is most often used to treat migraine headaches, an older set of drugs is still sometimes used. The three drugs in this group are ergotamine (Ergomar), a combination of ergotamine and caffeine (Cafergot), and a combination of dihydroergotamine and caffeine (Migranal). You should not consume grapefruit and grapefruit juice if you use any of these drugs. Grapefruit increases drug availability and the likelihood of unpleasant side effects, such as vertigo and nausea.

If you are prescribed one of these drugs, you should not use St. John's wort. The herbal supplement reduces the availability of the drug in the body and renders it *less* effective in treating a migraine attack.

## Nerve Pain Drugs

Neuropathic pain ("nerve pain") occurs when the nerve cells that send pain signals from the body to the spinal cord and brain are damaged. When these cells are damaged, they can become active and transmit signals when nothing is happening to the body that causes pain. The brain is getting a signal that pain is being experienced, but it is a false signal. Nerve damage can result from injury to a limb, diabetes, infections of the nerve cells, and cancer, among other things. And it's not just deep pain that is perceived. On the skin surface, which also gets signals from these damaged nerve cells, these false signals can lead not only to an experience of pain but also a feeling of numbness, tingling (pins and needles), itching, hot and cold sensations, and painful sensations from gentle stimulation (like a summer breeze or when the skin is brushed by fabric).

Fortunately, there are drugs for treating neuropathic pain. These are pregabalin (Lyrica), gabapentin (Neurontin and Gralise), gabapentin enacarbil (Horizant), and certain antidepressants. All of these are thought to act by turning down the flow of pain information into the spinal cord and up into the brain.

## MEDICATIONS FOR TREATING NERVE PAIN

Pregabalin (Lyrica®)
Gabapentin (Neurontin®, Gralise®)
Gabapentin enacarbil (Horizant®)
Some Antidepressants (Tricyclics, SNRIs)

Pregabalin (Lyrica) can be taken with or without food. This drug can cause drowsiness and dizziness, so alcohol should be avoided or used with extreme caution because it can enhance these feelings. Some herbal supplements, such as kava and valerian, also cause drowsiness and sleepiness. It is best to discontinue the use of both of these while using pregabalin, to avoid boosting this side effect.

Gabapentin (Neurontin, Gralise) can be taken without regard to food. But because food increases the absorption of Gralise, take it the same way every day. Gabapentin is often taken with dinner because it causes drowsiness. Avoid taking antacids containing magnesium and aluminum with gabapentin. The antacid reduces the absorption and availability of the drug, so take gabapentin at least two hours after the last ingestion of an antacid. Drowsiness is also a common side effect of gabapentin use. Avoid or greatly limit alcohol intake, because alcohol enhances drowsiness. All herbal supplements that cause drowsiness and sleepiness—like kava and valerian—should be discontinued if you are taking this drug.

**FOODS AND SUPPLEMENTS TO AVOID WHEN TAKING NERVE PAIN MEDICATIONS**

Alcohol
Kava
Valerian

Gabapentin enacarbil (Horizant) should be taken with food. If you are taking this drug, avoid consuming alcohol because it may increase the absorption and availability of the drug to the body, increasing the intensity of side effects. This drug causes dizziness and drowsiness, so in addition to avoiding alcohol, you should discontinue the use of any herbal supplements that cause drowsiness and sleepiness, especially kava and valerian.

A number of antidepressant drugs have been found to be helpful in treating some types of neuropathic pain. Several tricyclic antidepressants and SNRIs are used for this purpose. (See chapter 1 for information on the interaction of these drugs with food, nutrients, and supplements.)

## PATIENT STORY: ELIZABETH

Elizabeth had a high-powered job as a public relations executive. She loved her work, although she admitted lots of "crisis management" was involved almost daily. It was a high-stress position, but she felt she managed it well, and her health was basically fine. She was at a healthy weight, considered herself a healthy eater, and walked close to an hour every day. She seemed to have headaches more often than other people, but usually just took a few ibuprofens to get through the day.

More recently, she experienced headaches so severe she needed to take a sick day from work. She was sensitive to light and found some relief lying quietly in a darkened room. These headaches were debilitating for a day or two. She consulted a neurologist for advice, and the diagnosis was migraine headache. In a discussion of lifestyle issues with her doctor that might contribute to the migraines, Elizabeth felt her stressful job, as well as her overall lack of sleep, triggered them. She estimated she slept about five to six hours a night (healthy guidelines are seven to eight hours).

Her neurologist helped her understand that, while triggers can contribute to an episode, they don't directly cause them. She was prescribed a trial of eletriptan (Relpax). Elizabeth also agreed to work on stress management and on getting more sleep. A friend suggested she try meditation, and she found an app that helped her change her response to stress, as she agreed her job wasn't going to get less stressful. She also bumped up her sleep regularly to six to seven hours most nights, and eight hours at least twice a week. Her Relpax trial was a success. She tolerated the medicine well, it took less than two hours for some relief, and her sensitivity to light was greatly reduced.

While medication did not prevent a migraine, it surely managed her symptoms. Elizabeth gets a huge amount of relief from the medication, but also works on lifestyle habits under her control to help reduce the likelihood of future episodes.

## PATIENT STORY: HARRY

Harry is a type 2 diabetic, and was diagnosed about 16 years ago. At first he managed his condition with oral medications and adhered to his doctor's advice to lose some weight. Harry knew he could stand to lose about 30 pounds, but his doctor told him to "start small" and aim for just 10 percent of his starting weight, about 18 pounds. Even with this more modest goal, he struggled with his weight but was compliant in taking his medications; his blood sugar and A1C levels were stable and normal.

About a year ago, Harry needed to switch to insulin injections to manage his blood sugar. Now, after close to two decades with diabetes, Harry visited his doctor with complaints of severe leg pain for the past several months, which kept him up at night. His doctor explained he was experiencing the effects of nerve damage in his legs caused by the diabetes. Harry was prescribed Neurontin (gabapentin) for the pain. His doctor was right—his nightly pains were relieved. He was surprised to learn that he needed to avoid taking antacids at the same time he took Neurontin, because the antacid interfered with the action of the pain medication. Harry made sure to take the gabapentin at least two hours after taking the last antacid. And because the gabapentin might make him drowsy, his doctor suggested taking this in the evening. While Harry was not happy to be taking an additional medication, this pain relief was a great help. And it's now motivated him to try to eat healthier and get more activity to support a healthy lifestyle. With a better night's sleep, his quality of life has also improved.

# Chapter 3
# BLOOD THINNERS
# (Anticoagulants)

Blood thinner drugs include anticoagulants, platelet aggregation inhibitors, and drugs for treating peripheral vascular disease.

## *How Blood Thinners Work*

While this group of medicines is commonly referred to as "blood thinners," that term conjures up a strange image for most people. It's not a case of your blood becoming "watered down." While it might make visual sense to imagine that your blood is "thinner," making it easier to circulate through blood vessels all over your body, that's not what these medicines do. They instead act to block the creation of unwanted blood clots that can form even as blood flows normally through the blood vessels.

The truth is, the formation of blood clots in the body is normal, and quite necessary for blood vessel repair. However, when these clots go "renegade" and start forming when they shouldn't, or break off and circulate through the bloodstream, they can be life threatening. Your doctor might prescribe a blood thinner for you for a number of different medical reasons, but they are all connected to problems of excess blood clot formation. Don't be surprised if your friend or relative is taking the same blood thinner as you, but for a very different ailment. The end result for every person prescribed blood thinners is the same: to prevent an unwanted blood clot, while still allowing the body to form the *right* kind of clots, as needed, for everyday injury repairs. It's the unwanted clots that must be prevented. A bad clot might stop the flow of blood into an organ, depriving it of oxygen and nutrients. As a result, the organ may be damaged.

The good news is that these medications are very effective over many years in preventing unwanted blood clots from forming—assuming the medication is taken daily, and attention is paid to the diet. This is a case where daily food intake monitoring is essential, to enable the medication to take proper action. And it all comes down to a handful of nutrients: foods that contain vitamin K, for example, have a major impact on the effectiveness of a major blood thinner. There are other foods and supplements, too, and in this chapter we help you sort through your personal food choices as well as enable you to start an open dialogue with your doctor or nutritionist so you can be a smart eater while taking a blood thinner.

Before thinking about foods to avoid when taking blood thinners, you should understand a little bit about what these medicines do, and why the diet has a major impact on them—much more than many other medication types. The daily dosage of a blood thinner is carefully set to mimic the normal balance of blood clotting in the body—not too much and not too little. Once this balancing dose has been established for you, certain dietary choices can easily push you off this "sweet spot," making your blood likely to form too many or too few clots for normal body function.

Sometimes people are surprised to learn that the clotting of blood is a normal, protective action of the body. Think of the occasional cut you get; some bleeding occurs, and then it stops. That's a simple example of a blood clot *forming on the surface of your body.* A scab forms (nature's Band-Aid®), your skin heals underneath, and the scab falls off. Can you imagine a similar process occurring *inside* your body?

Here's what happens:

Normally, if a blood vessel gets a small tear, the body's natural defenses jump in, blocking the flow of blood out of the blood vessel into the surrounding tissue. Blood belongs *inside* our arteries and veins, not in the space outside of them. The body forms a clot—a biological Band-Aid on the inside of the blood vessel at the site of the breakage. The essential ingredients for forming a clot are already circulating in the blood. (The human body is amazing!)

One of these ingredients is small particles called "platelets," which team up with a series of specialized molecules to form a tough, fibrous mass. When a blood vessel breaks and the underlying tissue is exposed directly to the blood, some of the cells at the break site release molecules that attract platelets and cause them to form a little "plug." This starts a whole series of signals from the platelets and the cells surrounding the tear, causing them to grab molecules of fibrinogen (a protein) from the blood and modify them to create the tough matrix of the final blood clot.

During the body's natural healing process, as the clot blocks blood loss at the site of the tear, the surrounding tissue repairs the damaged blood vessel and gradually dissolves the clot when the tear is healed. The breakdown of the clot—as it is no longer needed—is activated by another compound already embedded in the clot. This is the step most similar to a scab falling off a cut on the surface of your body.

You may still be wondering, if blood clotting is a normal part of blood vessel repair, why do some people need to take medications to prevent clot formation? The key feature of the normal process is that it is restricted to sites where it is needed, such as the site of a blood vessel break. Here, the natural repair mechanism makes perfect sense. But there are several important blood constituents that *prevent the spread of the clot into the blood* as it flows past the site of the break. This prevention step is very important because, otherwise, clots would spread throughout the circulation. If that happened, those circulating clots would clog blood vessels all over the body, leading to very serious health consequences.

In certain disease states, clot formation can occur within the blood as it circulates, or clots can break off from repair sites, leading to strokes (blood vessel blockage by clots in the brain) and pulmonary emboli (blockage of blood vessels by clots in the lungs). Both are life-threatening situations. To prevent such fatal results with diseases that increase the occurrence of uncontrolled blood clot formation, drugs are regularly prescribed to reduce the likelihood of clot formation in the circulation. These drugs act to reduce the ability of a clot to form by diminishing the action of platelets or fibrin.

The two classes of blood thinners work differently, depending on what part of the clot-forming process they target, but the solution is the same: blocking excess clot formation. Diseases and conditions where these drugs may be prescribed include deep vein thrombosis (DVT), pulmonary embolism, angina, atrial fibrillation, myocardial infarction (heart attack), coronary artery bypass surgery, and surgical stent placement.

There are two different categories of drugs (taken by mouth) that inhibit clot formation: anticoagulants and platelet aggregation inhibitors. While both are linked together in the blood thinner category, they act very differently in the body. These two groups are typically divided by the kind of blood vessel that is targeted: veins, which operate at *low pressure* with blood flowing slowly, and arteries, which operate at *high pressure* with blood flowing very quickly.

The anticoagulants are used primarily to treat and prevent clot formation in slow-moving blood areas of the circulation, including the veins in the legs, in portions of the heart into which large veins empty (the atria), and in blood pooled behind natural and artificial heart valves. The diseases often associated with anticoagulant use include atrial fibrillation, deep vein thrombosis (DVT), pulmonary embolism, and the presence of artificial heart valves.

The platelet aggregation inhibitors are usually used both to treat and prevent clot formation in arteries, where blood normally moves quickly under high pressure. They are used in conditions including stroke and transient ischemic attack (TIA) in brain arteries (TIAs occur when small arteries contract temporarily, briefly reducing blood flow to a portion of the brain), acute coronary syndrome and coronary artery disease, and in peripheral artery disease affecting circulation in the lower body and legs. Some platelet aggregation inhibitors are used in combination with aspirin.

## *Medication Groups That Prevent Blood Clots*

Currently in the United States, two main medication groups are used to prevent blood clot formation: anticoagulants and platelet aggregation inhibitors. As described above, the manner in which the two groups block the formation of unwanted blood clots differs, but they are classified under the same general treatment umbrella of "blood thinners."

There are three main *anticoagulants* approved for use in the United States: warfarin (Coumadin®, Jantoven®), dabigatran (Pradaxa®), and rivaroxaban (Xarelto®).

The main *platelet aggregation inhibitors* are dipyridamole (Persantine®), clopidogrel (Plavix®), prasugrel (Effient®), and ticagrelor (Brilinta®). And it might surprise you to know that another platelet aggregation inhibitor is the well-known, over-the-counter product: aspirin!

**BLOOD THINNER MEDICATION GROUPS**

Anticoagulants:
- Warfarin (Coumadin, Jantoven)
- Dabigatran (Pradaxa)
- Rivaroxaban (Xarelto)

Platelet aggregation inhibitors:
- Dypyridamole (Persantine)
- Clopidogrel (Plavix)
- Prasugrel (Effient)
- Ticagrelor (Brilinta)
- Aspirin (generic); nonprescription

## Foods and Nutritional Supplements That Affect Anticoagulants and Platelet Aggregation Inhibitors

Although there are food and nutritional supplement interactions that are specific for *individual* blood thinners, some interactions pertain to *all*. It's important to remember that, while these drugs can prevent renegade clot formation in the circulation, *there is a fine line between preventing undesired clot formation and preventing all clot formation*. We do *not* want to prevent *all* clot formation; we need normal clotting to enable repair of damaged blood vessels (such as after a cut, or when we receive a blow that causes bruising). The goal is to prevent the excessive tendency to form clots that can occur in certain diseases.

Because of this sensitive balance in maintaining normal blood clotting throughout the body, if you have been prescribed any of these drugs, you'll be routinely asked to get blood work. This is to ensure you're taking enough medicine to block excessive clot formation (good), but not too much to block all clot formation (not good). The drug dose that achieves this careful balance will be unique to you, and will definitely be influenced by some of the foods and nutritional supplements you consume in your diet. These foods and supplements can either raise or lower your ability to form clots, which then changes the potency of the drug.

The first step before you begin taking a blood thinner is to show your doctor a list of the relevant foods you eat daily and how much you eat of each. You will also include on that list *all* vitamin and herbal supplements you take. Your doctor will work with you to make necessary dietary adjustments to ensure that the drug will provide a safe and consistent level of protection against excess clot formation. You may be asked to avoid certain foods and supplements completely, or to cut back on some foods. *Most importantly, you'll want to eat these foods in about the same amounts from week to week.* Consistency in your daily eating habits is especially important when taking blood thinners.

Be aware that your doctor will continue to ask you at each visit if you are following your diet *consistently*, and if there have been any changes since your last visit. He or she will be especially concerned if your blood test shows a change in clotting ability since your last visit. If a change has occurred, your doctor will need to know of any alterations in your diet to identify the correct source of the change in clotting ability and correct it. (It might or might not be due to a dietary change.)

## Adjusting Your Diet for Foods and Supplements That Affect Blood Thinners

**Vitamin E:** This vitamin can have modest anticoagulant action on its own, but only in *extremely* high doses—much higher than would be consumed in the normal diet. Our requirement for vitamin E is very small (around 15 mg daily, the amount in a standard multivitamin), and it's easy to meet those needs daily in everyday eating. It is very rare to have a vitamin E deficiency, but large amounts taken as a vitamin supplement can interfere with blood clotting.

Millions of people take vitamin E supplements because of the antioxidant action—we're told it is good for treating anything from diabetes to Alzheimer's disease. And for many people, when it comes to vitamins, they mistakenly think that more must be better. This is a big mistake when it comes to individuals taking blood thinners. It's essential to tell your doctor if you take a vitamin

E supplement (and the amount) when you *begin* treatment with a blood thinner. And if you're already taking a blood thinner, do not add a vitamin E supplement without first talking to your doctor. The large amounts of vitamin E in some supplements might alter the potency of the anticoagulant medicine you are taking.

> Vitamin E in supplement form (not foods) should be avoided when taking blood thinners.

**Omega-3 fatty acids (fish oils):** Eating fish regularly generally poses no health risk in terms of omega-3 fatty acids, even for people taking blood thinners, and provides multiple health benefits. But consuming the very large amounts of these fatty acids found in some fish-oil supplements can interfere with the effectiveness of blood thinner medications. The ingestion of fish oil or supplements containing omega-3 fatty acids may be sufficient to increase the antiplatelet and anticoagulant actions of the drugs you are taking, which would make bleeding more likely. Hence, be sure to tell your doctor if you are using these supplements. You may be asked to reduce your intake of them.

> Fish oils in supplement form should be avoided when taking blood thinners. However, eating fish is OK.

**Onions and garlic:** While onion and garlic both contain compounds that can act like a blood thinner, it only becomes a concern when these are consumed in very large amounts. Typical daily intake of these compounds from foods is not a health risk. However, if you consume huge amounts of onions or garlic daily, you might increase the risk of bleeding. And this is particularly true of garlic supplements, which would concentrate the amount of garlic acting on your body. Remember to check with your doctor for personalized advice.

---

Avoid garlic supplements and large amounts of garlic or onions in foods.

---

In addition to these broad dietary considerations, there are additional food and nutrient issues that apply only to one or the other drug class (anticoagulants, platelet aggregation inhibitors):

Anticoagulants (warfarin [Coumadin®, Jantoven®], dabigatran [Pradaxa®], rivaroxaban [Xarelto®]): These drugs can all be taken with or without food. However, there are many items you consume in your diet that can influence how well these drugs work in your body. We have already discussed the importance of moderating your consumption of onion, garlic, and certain supplements (vitamin E, omega-3 fatty acids/fish oil). At the present time, other food items suspected or known to influence the actions of anticoagulant drugs have been studied mostly for warfarin. The suspicion is that these food items may also apply to the other anticoagulants.

So for the time being, it is best to be cautious, and apply the information available for warfarin to the other anticoagulant drugs. The food items to be avoided include alcoholic beverages, soy milk, pomegranate, cranberries, green tea (only when consumed in large amounts— more than 32 ounces/day), mango and avocado. For rivaroxaban [Xarelto®] only, the ingestion of grapefruit and grapefruit juice should be limited (one-half a grapefruit or 6–8 ounces of grapefruit juice each day) or avoided. Since you may include one or more of these foods in your diet, and vary which ones you eat from day to day, the best approach is to reduce how much you consume of each, or even better, to eliminate them from your diet, if possible. Above all, remember to be consistent from week to week in how much of these foods you choose to eat, if you retain them in your diet.

For warfarin alone, there is one other very important nutritional issue, vitamin K. Vitamin K is a required ingredient in the formation of a blood clot. Once it is used for this purpose, it becomes inactive, and the active form must be regenerated. Warfarin slows the regeneration process, thereby reducing the active form of vitamin K and thus the overall ability of the body to form clots. If you eat foods containing lots of vitamin K, you will increase the amount of active vitamin K in blood (dietary vitamin K is in the active form), and thus reduce the level of anticoagulation produced by warfarin. That's why the total amount of vitamin K in the diet is so important, and also why you need to eat consistent amounts of vitamin K on a daily or weekly basis.

Vitamin K intake in the diet is a two-part issue if you take warfarin: you want to keep the total amount of vitamin K you consume in your diet on the low side, and you want to consume roughly the same amount of vitamin K in your diet from day to day. Remember that there is a definite, daily requirement of vitamin K that must be met for good health (even while you are taking a blood thinner). If you take a multivitamin or mineral supplement, on the label you'll find a recommended dietary allowance (RDA) or daily value. The RDA for vitamin K is around 90 micrograms (mcg) for women and 120 mcg for men. Translated into food, this means less than one serving of a dark-green, leafy vegetable typically meets your daily vitamin K requirement (these vegetables contain 100–400 mcg per serving). So there's little risk of vitamin K deficiency if you cut back on your intake when you're taking blood thinners.

If you're a big salad and green vegetable eater, it's very important to talk to your doctor about cutting back your intake as needed, to keep your medication dosage on target. This is not an exact science, but mindfulness of daily eating is particularly important when you are taking warfarin. If you take a multivitamin or mineral supplement, make sure to include it when estimating your daily intake of vitamin K, and avoid high-potency vitamins that may contain extra vitamin K. Similar to foods with vitamin K, your multivitamin or mineral supplement must be taken *daily* for consistency.

Review your diet to look for foods rich in vitamin K: collard greens, spinach, salad greens, broccoli, Brussels sprouts, cabbage, and Bibb lettuce. Anywhere from 100 to 300 mcg of vitamin K consumed from these vegetables daily should be fine. (See table 1 on page 71 for serving sizes.) Notice that soybean and canola oils also contain significant amounts of the vitamin.

## TABLE 1. FOODS CONTAINING HIGH AMOUNTS OF VITAMIN K

*Note:* Watch out for the foods below when taking warfarin.

| Food | Amount | Vitamin K Content (mcg) |
|------|--------|-------------------------|
| Brussels sprouts | 1 cup | 300 |
| Broccoli | 1 cup | 220 |
| Collard greens | 1 cup | 775 |
| Cabbage or coleslaw | 1 cup | 165 |
| Canola oil | 4 tablespoons | 60 |
| Endive | 1 cup chopped | 115 |
| Kale | 1 cup chopped | 1100 |
| Lettuce* (Bibb or red leaf) | 1 cup chopped | 105 |
| Soybean oil | 4 tablespoons | 100 |
| Spinach | 1 cup cooked | 900 |

*Dark-green, leafy vegetables are all rich sources of vitamin K. If your favorite green is not listed here, use the lettuce amount as your guide.

⬤ If you take warfarin, determine your total daily vitamin K intake. Keep it adequate for good health (the RDA amount) but otherwise as low as possible, and ingest roughly the same amount every day while taking warfarin. A healthy, safe range is 100–300 mcg daily, but talk to your doctor when taking blood thinners to agree on the right amount for you that you can stick to consistently—without a struggle. This is particularly true for those who are big salad eaters!

Platelet aggregation inhibitors (dipyridamole [Persantine®], clopidogrel [Plavix®], prasugrel [Effient®], and ticagrelor [Brilinta®]): These drugs may be taken with or without food, *except* for dipyridamole [Persantine®], which should be taken two hours before or after a meal (because food affects the drug's absorption into the body). For these foods, there is only one other food concern (other than the general concerns discussed above for all blood thinners): if you eat grapefruit or grapefruit juice, limit your intake to one-half a grapefruit or one 6–8-ounce glass of grapefruit juice each day for all of the platelet aggregation inhibitors *except* dipyridamole [Persantine®]. Grapefruit alters the bioavailability of these drugs in the body.

Because the dietary (and nutritional supplement) issues are complex, it is best to discuss this issue carefully with your doctor, who may also refer you to a registered dietician for a personalized dietary plan.

## *Herbal Supplements That Modify the Effects of Blood Thinner Drugs*

A number of herbal supplements are known to increase or decrease the potency of antiplatelet and anticoagulant drugs. *Many more probably exist, for which these effects are not yet known.* It is essential to discuss with your doctor *all* of the herbal supplements you take before you begin to use anticoagulant or antiplatelet drugs. You will probably be asked to stop taking *all* supplements known to have effects on bleeding, and perhaps others that you take. As explained earlier, there is a fine line for medication dosage between the beneficial effects and the undesirable side effects of these drugs. Producers of herbal supplements are not required by law to identify the active ingredients they contain. *The safest approach when using antiplatelet and anticoagulant drugs is to discontinue the use of all herbal supplements while taking these medicines.*

At present, the herbal supplements most commonly thought to influence the ability of the *anticoagulants* to work in your body are American and Asian ginseng, ginkgo biloba, ginger, saw palmetto, St. John's wort, danshen, dong quai, boldo and lycium barbarum. The herbal supplements most commonly thought to influence the ability of the platelet aggregation inhibitors to work in your body are ginkgo biloba, Asian ginseng, bilberry, ginger, horse chestnut, and (for ticagrelor [Brilinta®] only) St. John's wort.

## DIETARY SUPPLEMENT ALERT!

**Herbal (Dietary) Supplements to Avoid When Taking Blood Thinner Medications:**

With anticoagulant drugs:
- American or Asian ginseng
- Ginger
- Ginkgo biloba
- Saw palmetto
- St. John's wort
- Danshen
- Dong quai
- Boldo
- Lycium barbarum

With antiplatelet drugs:
- Ginkgo biloba
- Asian ginseng
- Bilberry
- Ginger
- Horse chestnut
- St. John's wort (*Ticagrelor only*)

## FOODS AND VITAMIN SUPPLEMENTS TO LIMIT OR AVOID WHEN TAKING BLOOD THINNER MEDICATIONS

Foods containing vitamin K (*Warfarin only*):
- Collard greens
- Spinach
- Salad greens
- Broccoli
- Brussels sprouts
- Cabbage
- Bibb lettuce

Garlic (large amounts)
Onion (large amounts)

Cooking oils:
- Soybean oil
- Canola oil

Supplements:
- Vitamin E supplements (the amount in foods is not risky)
- Fish oil supplements (the amount in fish is not risky)
- Omega-3 fatty acids (may be present in some multi-component dietary supplements [read ingredients labels carefully])

*Note:* Keep your intake of these foods and vitamins consistent from day to day — always talk to your doctor about any changes in your intake of them.

## ADDITIONAL FOOD RESTRICTIONS FOR BLOOD THINNERS

Avoid the following foods for anticoagulants:
- Soy milk (limit to 8 ounces)
- Pomegranate juice (limit to 8 ounces)
- Cranberry juice (limit to 8 ounces)
- Grapefruit juice (limit to 8 ounces) or grapefruit (limit to one-half grapefruit)
- Green tea (limit to 32 ounces a day)
- Mango
- Avocado
- Alcoholic beverages

Avoid grapefruit and grapefruit juice for the following platelet aggregation inhibitors:
- Clopidogrel (Plavix)
- Prasugrel (Effient)
- Ticagrelor (Brilinta)

## PATIENT STORY: BARBARA

Barbara, 50 years old, was told by her doctor that she would be taking a blood thinner as part of her treatment for atrial fibrillation to ameliorate the risk of developing dangerous blood clots. A self-described "clean eater" and at a healthy weight, Barbara was upset when she thought that she would need to cut out all salads and dark-green, leafy vegetables, as she had heard. She worried about her weight and the impact of such a major dietary change. She wanted to be healthy, but what would she eat?

Barbara was relieved to learn that it was not necessary to cut out all of her dark-green, leafy vegetables and salads. The most important thing, as she learned, was to *maintain* the same amount of greens in her daily eating. Working with her doctor, she planned to eat two small salads daily—about two cups worth—and her medication was adjusted accordingly, to work with that amount of extra vitamin K from her diet. Her doctor further explained that she couldn't binge on salads and then skip them for a few days. She needed to keep the overall amount of salad she was eating roughly the same from day to day. Barbara understood clearly that her vitamin K intake needed to remain stable every day.

With this new mindset, Barbara was set up for success in maintaining a normal diet that she enjoyed and found it much easier to comply with the instructions for the medication. She remains active and weight stable, enjoying the foods she loves—in moderation and consistency. A definite win-win!

## PATIENT STORY: MARK

Mark had been under the care of a cardiologist for many years, knowing he had a congenital valve problem in his heart. His doctor prescribed a blood thinner to prevent blood clots from forming on the damaged valve. During his yearly examination, they reviewed his diet, medicines, and supplements, and his doctor pointed out to Mark that certain foods and supplements might interfere with his blood thinner. He'd been taking ginger as a supplement as well as ginkgo biloba in the hope of boosting his energy and vitality, and perhaps his memory. Mark was surprised to hear that these two supplements, which he thought would help his health, would have to be discontinued during the blood thinner therapy.

Clearly understanding the risks of taking these supplements with a blood thinner, Mark decided discontinuing the supplements was a no-brainer. Instead of taking them, he exercises regularly (an hour-long, brisk walk daily) for an energy boost and found an online game app to improve his mindfulness and mental focus.

# Chapter 4
# DIABETES MEDICINES

Medications to treat diabetes fall into two main categories: drugs that must be injected and those that are taken by mouth. Insulin is the best-known injectable "drug" (actually a hormone) for treating diabetes. There are other hormones that are also given by injection that act to enhance the normally occurring insulin secretion of the body. Medications are given by injection to bypass the stomach and intestines, and thus avoid many of the issues and problems that arise when medicines are consumed along with foods and dietary supplements. As these latter issues are central to this book, our discussion here is limited to diabetes medications that are taken by mouth, pass along the digestive tract, and are absorbed.

If you take insulin, of course, there are important issues relating to when injections should be given in relation to consuming foods. These details must be worked out carefully between you and your doctor, and include monitoring of your blood sugar level to make sure it does not fall too low when you give yourself an injection. We do not discuss them here.

Your doctor will also help you to adjust your overall diet to harmonize with your type of diabetes and treatment plan. Further guidance on foods to eat when you have diabetes is available from many other healthcare professionals, including registered dieticians, and from diabetes-focused organizations, such as the American Diabetes Association.

Knowing what diabetes actually means is essential to understanding how foods can affect the action of drugs taken orally to treat the disease. Diabetes is a chronic disease that occurs when your body fails to handle efficiently the sugars and other carbohydrates you consume in your diet each day. There are many dietary sources of sugars and carbohydrates. Foods naturally contain "simple" sugars (such as fructose in fruits, or sucrose in sugar cane and sugar beets) that your taste buds sense as having a sweet flavor. There are also "complex carbohydrates," also known as starches, that are found in breads, rice, pasta, potatoes, cereals, and other grains. Complex carbohydrates are very long chains of simple sugars linked together that don't taste particularly sweet. While these sugars occur naturally in foods, there are also "added sugars" and "added carbohydrates,"—simple sugars that are added to a boxed or packaged product to *increase* their sweetness, or complex carbohydrates that are added to increase bulk and firmness.

The biological reality is that *when it comes to added sugars, the body sees them metabolically as all the same!* This means that adding brown sugar, honey, agave, molasses, or any other source of sugar to food is no better (or worse) than adding white table sugar, known as sucrose. By and large, the body handles all of these sugars the same way.

Once consumed, your stomach and intestines digest these sugars and complex carbohydrates, breaking them down into their simplest units: glucose, fructose, and galactose. The most basic by-products of dietary sugars and complex carbohydrates, they can be readily absorbed by your intestines and transferred into the blood. Once in the bloodstream, they circulate throughout the body and are absorbed by all cells. They are used to make energy, powering all life functions.

But sugars can't normally enter a cell very quickly on their own. To stimulate this process, they require insulin.

Insulin is made in the pancreas and released into blood in response to increases in blood sugar levels, which normally occur when you eat and drink. The insulin released when you eat circulates throughout the body and directly signals to the cells that it's time to take up sugars from the bloodstream. When the cells absorb the sugars, the blood sugar drops back again to the normal resting level.

Diabetes is a condition that occurs in two different ways. The first is when the pancreas cannot produce and release insulin, a disease called "type 1" diabetes (sometimes referred to as "childhood" diabetes). In type 1 diabetes, insulin injections are given with meals to provide the missing hormone. Insulin cannot be taken orally, because it is destroyed in the stomach and intestines. So it must be injected to bypass the digestive tract.

The second form of diabetes is "type 2" diabetes (previously called "adult onset" diabetes), which is much more prevalent than type 1—affecting children, teens, and adults. In type 2 diabetes, the cells in your body respond sluggishly to the insulin released from the pancreas, and blood sugar remains high much longer after a meal than is normal. Type 2 diabetes most often develops as a result of obesity. The pancreas responds by releasing more insulin, which helps for a while, but eventually drug intervention becomes necessary to keep blood sugar levels down. The good news is that weight loss—even losing 10 percent of your starting weight—can often resolve type 2 diabetes without the use of medication.

In *both* types of diabetes, blood sugar levels in your blood become abnormally high during most of the day and night, which is not a healthy thing. If you're wondering why high blood sugar is a problem for the body, the reason is that the sugars in your blood will begin to react with other body components, like proteins. When this excess sugar comes in contact with proteins, enzymes, and other compounds, it damages them, reducing their ability to carry out their normal functions. Over time, if not corrected, this process causes many of the problems associated with diabetes, including damage to the kidneys and its blood vessels, vision problems, nervous system problems in the legs and elsewhere, and various cardiovascular issues. Without treatment, diabetes is eventually life threatening.

The goal in treating diabetes is to restore the body's ability to efficiently handle the flow of sugars through the blood after a meal so that they are rapidly taken up by cells, and blood sugar levels quickly return to baseline levels. This process greatly reduces the chance of any sugar-related damage to body cells. When the pancreas no longer makes insulin and you're diagnosed with type 1 diabetes, the usual treatment is insulin injection.

If the pancreas can still make insulin but the cells in the body are less responsive to it (type 2 diabetes), oral medications can be used to restore the ability of your cells to respond to insulin. One class of drugs acts by boosting insulin secretion from the pancreas, so it squirts out more in response to rising blood sugar levels. Another class of medicines increases the sensitivity of body cells to insulin, so less insulin can be more effective in stimulating them to absorb sugars from blood. Yet another class of drugs simply *slows* the speed at which sugar molecules are digested and absorbed from the intestines. Spreading absorption out over a longer period of time keeps blood sugar lower. It is particularly important to blunt peak blood sugar levels after food or beverage ingestion, to prevent dangerously high levels. Depending on how far your disease has progressed, your physician may use one or more of these drugs.

## MEDICATIONS FOR TREATING TYPE 2 DIABETES

Medications that slow sugar digestion and absorption from the intestines:
- Acarbose (Precose®)
- Miglitol (Glyset®)

Medications that *directly* enhance insulin release from the pancreas:
- Glimepiride (Amaryl®)
- Glipizide (Glucotrol®, Glucotrol XL®)
- Glyburide (Diabeta®, Glynase Pres-Tab®)
- Nateglinide (Starlix®)
- Repaglinide (Prandin®)

Medications that *indirectly* enhance insulin release from the pancreas:
- Alogliptin (Nesina®)
- Linagliptin (Tradjenta®)
- Saxagliptin (Onglyza®)
- Sitagliptin (Januvia®)

Medications that enhance body cell sensitivity to insulin:
- Metformin (Glucophage®, Glumetza®, Riomet®, Fortamet®)
- Pioglitazone (Actos®)
- Rosiglitazone (Avandia®)

## *Type 2 Diabetes Drugs*

Research in drug development for diabetes has been very successful in creating a variety of medications that act in different ways to help regulate blood sugar. The treatment options for type 2 diabetes are many, and coupled with a healthy lifestyle—smart eating, physical activity, no smoking, and stress reduction—are a solid recipe for success. Understanding how these medications work in the body can help you understand *why* what you eat can affect the action of different drugs. There are many drugs to treat diabetes, with the common goal of keeping blood sugar levels in a lower, stable, and healthy range. Because they act in different ways, and are eliminated in different ways by the body, it's not surprising that their interactions with dietary and herbal supplements also differ.

### Types of Drugs

The medications that *slow sugar digestion and absorption* from the intestines are Miglitol (Glyset®) and Acarbose (Precose®). These drugs slow the release of digested sugars into the bloodstream from the intestines, blunting the rise in the blood sugar level that occurs during and after food ingestion.

Another set of drugs acts directly to *enhance the ability of the pancreas to release insulin* when blood sugar levels rise. These medications include Glimepiride (Amaryl), Glyburide (Diabeta, Glynase Pres-Tab), Glipizide (Glucotrol, Glucotrol XL), Repaglinide (Prandin), and Nateglinide (Starlix). The normal response of the body is to release insulin from the pancreas when blood sugar levels increase. This group of medications acts directly on the pancreas to boost the amount of insulin released in response to a rise in blood sugar. The more insulin that is released, the lower blood sugar levels rise.

Yet another group of drugs can enhance the ability of the pancreas to release insulin when blood sugar levels rise after a meal. But these drugs do not act *directly* on the pancreas, like those described above. They act by *elevating blood levels of another hormone (incretin) that in turn increases the sensitivity of the pancreas to blood sugar levels, and releases more insulin.* These drugs are Sitagliptin (Januvia®), Linagliptin (Tradjenta®), Saxagliptin (Onglyza®), and Alogliptin (Nesina®).

A final set of medications help to lower blood sugar levels by increasing the sensitivity of body cells to the effects of insulin. Essentially, these drugs act to make insulin have a *greater* effect on the cells so they absorb more sugar from the bloodstream. The net result is lower blood sugar levels. This group of medications includes metformin (Glucophage, Glumetza, Riomet, Fortamet), pioglitazone (Actos), and rosiglitazone (Avandia).

While each drug is discussed separately in this chapter, there are *four* important facts that apply to *all* drugs used to treat type 2 diabetes. The first is that using medications to treat diabetes is only one part of a comprehensive program for chronic management of this disease.

Both healthy food choices and regular exercise activities make important contributions to managing diabetes. For optimal management of your blood sugar levels, and to avoid the ailments often accompanying diabetes, it is important to follow *all* of the components of this comprehensive treatment program. The second point deals with the use of alcoholic beverages as a diabetic, the third with the use of nutritional and herbal supplements that may reduce blood sugar, and the fourth with the use of supplements that can raise blood sugar.

Because these latter points are central issues of this book, they are set out separately below.

## Guidelines for Consuming Foods and Supplements When Taking Type 2 Diabetes Drugs

**Alcohol:** *Alcohol consumption directly influences blood sugar levels.* Ingesting a moderately large amount of alcohol at a single occasion has the immediate effect of *reducing* blood sugar levels, while ingesting high amounts of alcohol on a regular basis *increases* blood sugar levels. Alcohol's effects are complicated. For most people with diabetes, alcohol does *not* have to be eliminated from the diet, but limiting daily intake to moderately low levels is very important. If you choose to consume alcohol, a conversation with your doctor is key, so that you understand *exactly* how much is safe. The government recommends limiting alcohol intake to no more than one daily drink for women, and two daily drinks for men. The serving size of "one drink" is 5 ounces of wine, 12 ounces of beer, or 1.5 ounces of hard spirits. Keep this in mind, as most people look at a serving as whatever is in the glass they are given! This is a particular problem at restaurants, where a "glass" of wine might have nearly double the standard serving size—which counts as two drinks.

Remember that if you ingest a level of alcohol that *lowers* your blood sugar levels, this may *increase* the effect of any drugs you are taking to reduce blood sugar. This can result in a blood sugar level that is dangerously *low* and cause dizziness and fainting. If you ingest large amounts of alcohol on a regular basis, which causes blood sugar to be high, the dose of medication you are taking may not keep your blood sugar level low enough. Over time, this results in elevated blood sugar levels that can increase the damage caused by the disease.

**FOODS TO LIMIT WHEN TAKING MEDICATIONS FOR TYPE 2 DIABETES**

**Alcohol**—occasional use; limit to one serving, which is 5 ounces of wine, 12 ounces of beer, or 1.5 ounces of hard spirits

**Grapefruit and grapefruit juice**—only for repaglinide and nateglinide; limit to one-half grapefruit or one 6–8-ounce glass of grapefruit juice daily

**Vitamins, minerals, and supplements advertised to lower blood sugar:** *Avoid these.* Many diabetics take a variety of supplements because of their advertised ability to lower blood sugar and help in treating diabetes. While these ads seem very appealing, they are *not* regulated for accuracy! When it comes to supplements claiming to lower blood sugar, if it sounds too good to be true, it probably is. The evidence that these supplements have such effects is very weak or lacking altogether. And in cases where evidence does exist, the effects are relatively small. The key take-home message is that when you have diabetes, you should *not* use such supplements as your only treatment, as they will *not* lower blood glucose levels into the normal (safe) range.

In addition, when you are taking a prescription drug to treat your diabetes, *do not* add a dietary supplement that is advertised to lower blood sugar without first consulting with your physician. Because the actions of these supplements are not well studied or documented, their actual effect on blood sugar levels can be uneven. *If a* supplement actually *does* lower blood sugar, when taken along with your prescription drug, the combination may lower blood sugar so low that you become dizzy and faint. And because dietary supplements are sold for a variety of ailments, you may be taking supplements for a condition unrelated to diabetes that might also lower blood sugar. Overall, if you are taking one or more diabetes prescription drugs, tell your doctor *whenever you think about adding* a supplement to your diet for *any* reason, to avoid an unexpected and unpleasant drop in blood sugar.

Dozens of oral supplements claim to lower blood sugar levels. A current list of some of the many compounds reputed to lower blood sugar includes agaricus mushroom, aloe vera, alpha-lipoic acid, American and Asian ginsengs, banaba, bean pod, blond psyllium, bitter melon, chia seeds, chromium picolinate, cinnamon, coenzyme Q10, fenugreek, glucomannan, guar gum, gymnema sylvestra, ivy gourd, magnesium, milk thistle, oat bran, prickly pear cactus, soy, stevia, and white mulberry. A good place to find out more about herbal and nutritional supplements that alter blood sugar is at the American Diabetes Association website ShopDiabetes.org. Select "Diabetes" from the menu at the top, then "eBooks" for "Guide to Herbs and Nutritional Supplements."

Two particular mineral supplements have been associated with lowering blood sugar: magnesium and chromium. Magnesium supplementation is thought to be helpful *only* in individuals who are magnesium deficient, something your doctor can determine with a blood test. The same is also thought to be true for chromium. If you take a multivitamin containing 100 percent of the recommended vitamin and mineral amounts every day, which includes chromium, you are unlikely to need more. Always check with your doctor.

# DIETARY SUPPLEMENT ALERT!

## Avoid These Supplements When Taking Oral Diabetes Medications:

Supplements that may lower blood sugar:
- Agaricus mushroom
- Aloe vera
- Alpha-lipoic acid
- American and Asian ginsengs
- Banaba
- Bean pod
- Blond psyllium
- Bitter melon
- Chia seeds
- Chromium picolinate
- Cinnamon
- Coenzyme Q10
- Fenugreek
- Glucomannan
- Guar gum
- Gymnema sylvestra
- Ivy gourd
- Magnesium
- Milk thistle
- Oat bran
- Prickly pear cactus
- Soy
- Stevia
- White mulberry

Supplements that can raise blood sugar:
- Nicotinic acid (niacin)—dose of three or more grams per day

St. John's wort makes the following drugs work less effectively:
- Nateglinide (Starlix)
- Repaglinide (Prandin)
- Linagliptin (Tradjenta)
- Saxagliptin (Onglyza)
- Pioglitazone (Actos)

**Dietary supplements:** *Some dietary supplements may also raise blood sugar.* Their use should be limited or avoided if you are diabetic. An example is nicotinic acid (niacin), when taken in high daily doses (more than 3,000 milligrams per day). Niacin is a B vitamin (an essential nutrient), so you must consume some each day. But the amount you need is quite small (around 20 milligrams per day), and does not affect blood sugar at this intake level. High daily doses of niacin are only given to some patients to help reduce high blood lipid levels and should occur only under the guidance of a physician.

## *Optimizing Your Medication: Timing of Doses with or without Food*

For the medications that help regulate blood sugar, there are almost no specific food and drug interactions (except for alcohol). Key factors in the effectiveness of antidiabetes medications are the *time* you take your medicine, and whether you need to take it *with or without food*. These guidelines vary, depending on how the medicine lowers blood sugar. As with all other medications, it's important to take the drug *as prescribed by your doctor*. Follow these guidelines for the antidiabetes drugs for optimal blood sugar regulation and ultimately to prevent your blood sugar levels from becoming too high, or too low.

**Drugs that slow sugar digestion and absorption:** For this drug class, including miglitol (Glyset) and acarbose (Precose), take your medication *just before a meal* for maximum effect. Limit your daily alcohol consumption as well as the use of dietary and herbal supplements on the basis of your doctor's recommendations.

**Drugs that directly enhance insulin release when blood sugar levels rise:** The drugs in this group are glimepiride (Amaryl), glyburide (Diabeta, Glynase Pres-Tab), glipizide (Glucotrol, Glucotrol XL), repaglinide (Prandin), and nateglinide (Starlix). These medications all need to be taken around mealtime, but not on an empty stomach because they release insulin, which lowers blood sugar levels. If you do not take them with a meal, blood sugar levels may fall enough to make you feel dizzy or faint. As with all antidiabetes drugs, limit daily alcohol consumption and the use of dietary and herbal supplements on the basis of your doctor's recommendations.

It's important to pay attention to when you take the drugs in this group in relation to food ingestion, because the timing is quite specific. If you take glimepiride (Amaryl) or glyburide (Diabeta, Glynase Pres-Tab), take your pill with the first meal of the day. If a second pill is prescribed to be taken later in the day, take with an additional meal. If you are taking glipizide (Glucotrol, Glucotrol XL), take the pill about 30 minutes before a meal.

*Magnesium-containing antacids* (read the label on the antacid bottle) can alter the effectiveness of some medications. If you take glimepiride (Amaryl), glyburide (Diabeta, Glynase Pres-Tab) or glipizide (Glucotrol, Glucotrol XL), do *not* take your pill at the same time you take an antacid. Take your pill at least two hours before or after you take the antacid. Magnesium increases how quickly your body absorbs these drugs and, if taken with the drug, could cause a larger than normal drop in blood glucose.

For repaglinide (Prandin) and nateglinide (Starlix), take pills *just before meals*. One further interaction to avoid if you take repaglinide (Prandin): if you eat grapefruit or drink grapefruit juice, limit your intake to either one-half grapefruit or one glass (6–8 ounces) of grapefruit juice each day, and avoid using St. John's wort. Both modify how quickly the body disposes of this drug and, in turn, alter how well the drug works to control your blood sugar levels. While grapefruit does *not* affect nateglinide (Starlix), St. John's wort needs to be avoided, as this supplement can change how well the medication works.

**Drugs that indirectly increase insulin release when blood sugar levels rise:** This drug group includes sitagliptin (Januvia), linagliptin (Tradjenta), saxagliptin (Onglyza), and alogliptin (Nesina). All of these drugs may be taken with or without food. As with the other categories, limit daily alcohol consumption and the use of dietary and herbal supplements on the basis of your doctor's recommendations. For *two* of these drugs—linagliptin (Tradjenta) and saxagliptin (Onglyza)—avoid using St. John's wort, as this supplement can interfere with their action.

**Drugs that enhance the sensitivity of cells to insulin:** While the drugs in this group act the same way to moderate blood sugar, each drug has a different optimal dosing regimen. Medications in this class include metformin (Glucophage, Glumetza, Riomet, Fortamet), pioglitazone (Actos), and rosiglitazone (Avandia).

For metformin, take your pills *with meals* to avoid stomach upset. Since metformin may decrease vitamin B12 levels in blood, these levels should be regularly monitored. If B12 levels are low, your doctor may recommend that you take a vitamin B12 supplement. A sublingual (under the tongue) form is often recommended because of better absorption by the body compared with a pill. Alternatively, your doctor may suggest monthly B12 injections.

You may take pioglitazone or rosiglitazone *with or without food* (in the morning for those who take one pill each day). For both of these drugs, limit daily alcohol consumption and the use of dietary and herbal supplements on the basis of your doctor's recommendations. For pioglitazone, specifically, you should avoid taking St. John's wort, as this supplement can interfere with the action of the drug.

## PATIENT STORY: VIVIAN

At the age of 42, Vivian was dismayed to see how her weight had crept up over the past 10 years. She'd had three children and always struggled with post-pregnancy weight loss. Her three pregnancies left her with an added 25 pounds—which continued to creep up over the past five years—leaving her with about 35 pounds to lose. She felt pretty good, although the added weight made her tired. But it was hard to know whether the tiredness came from a busy job and three daughters, or something else.

At her annual physical, Vivian's doctor (who had been concerned by her weight over the past few years) reviewed her laboratory work and told her she had developed type 2 diabetes. Her fasting blood sugar was elevated, as was her hemoglobin A1C level (an index of long-term blood sugar control). While she was shocked and frightened to hear this, her doctor assured her that a treatment plan including healthy eating, more physical activity, and some weight loss, along with medication, was effective and comprehensive.

Vivian was motivated to do her part and met with a nutritionist to develop a strategy for eating and activity that she could manage. For starters, she cut way back on her alcohol intake to make it moderate, limiting her consumption to a daily 5-ounce glass of wine. This was also an easy way to trim extra calories. She made time for a daily 30-minute walk. Her doctor prescribed metformin, a drug that boosted her body's ability to use insulin more effectively to lower her blood sugar. At first, she told her doctor that metformin did not agree with her, as she was having digestive problems. Then she discovered that taking her medication with meals resolved that problem easily, and she left her pill container on the kitchen table as a reminder.

Vivian's doctor had warned her that her vitamin B12 levels might drop with metformin treatment. When he measured B12 levels, at the same time he took the regular measurement of her fasting blood sugar levels, B12 was below normal. She was somewhat surprised, since she took a daily multivitamin. Her doctor suggested a B12 supplement, recommending the sublingual (under the tongue) form, which is more easily absorbed by the body.

Vivian's been feeling great, and the metformin treatment, because it supports better glucose-insulin balance, has made her weight loss effort a bit easier. Losing 10 pounds has been both a mental and physical boost to her health. She was thrilled when her doctor was able to decrease her daily dose of metformin because of her weight loss, diet, and exercise.

## PATIENT STORY: BRUCE

A busy executive, Bruce had been taking glipizide (Glucotrol) for about six months, had lost a few pounds, and was feeling much better. He especially liked the regularity of a daily treadmill walk to relieve workplace stress. The glipizide worked well for him, and his doctor confirmed that his blood sugar and A1C levels were in the normal range. But, wondering if the dose of the medication was too strong, Bruce called his doctor. Recently, he'd been experiencing some bouts of feeling slightly faint, and a little bit dizzy. He shrugged it off at first but, after a few episodes, made the call to his doctor.

It turned out that Bruce had been doing a lot of business travel and was outside of his typical lifestyle structure. He often found himself taking his medication upon awakening—on an empty stomach—so he didn't forget. He had good intentions, but taking glipizide on an empty stomach can make it work too well—and likely lower blood sugar too much, resulting in the symptoms Bruce experienced. Bruce now understands that he must always take this medication shortly before a meal, so there is food in his stomach and intestines, and sugars being absorbed, when the drug begins to lower blood sugar.

A second, controllable factor also likely to have contributed to his symptoms was Bruce's chronic acid reflux, for which he often took antacids throughout the day. He knew that losing more weight would likely help with the acid reflux but relied on antacids to relieve his symptoms. He hadn't noticed that his dizziness and a fainting feeling coincided with his taking the glipizide along with the antacid.

Many antacids contain magnesium (including Bruce's brand), which can amplify the effect of glipizide. Magnesium boosts the drug's absorption by the intestines, resulting in a larger-than-normal drop in blood sugar. When Bruce became mindful of this combination and avoided taking an antacid with his glipizide—allowing at least two hours to pass before taking an antacid—his symptoms went away.

# Chapter 5
# HEARTBURN (Acid Reflux) MEDICINES

At one time or another, nearly everyone experiences a bout or two of indigestion or heartburn. Both are generally recognizable—and universally understood—to reflect that sense of burning (sometimes pain) in the middle of your chest after eating. While heartburn and indigestion are only an occasional inconvenience for some people, millions struggle with recurring symptoms of this burning feeling. Later in the chapter, we discuss the importance of recognizing these symptoms and seeking medical advice, but it's important to know that what you might sense as chronic indigestion might be symptoms of something more. Symptoms of heartburn—more accurately called "acid reflux"—might also be symptoms of heart disease. And even if your diagnosis is definitively acid reflux, the visit to your doctor is important; as the medications treating this disorder vary, you'll want to get personalized professional advice.

## Acid Reflux

The term "acid reflux" is familiar to many and provides a big clue as to *why* you experience a burning sensation after eating. The reason is excess stomach acid. While it might sound scary that acid is part of food digestion, it makes sense when you consider that foods need to be broken down in the stomach into a digestible form. Controlled amounts of acid, released by the stomach in response to food, help achieve this. When the normal signals get out of whack, there's too much acid, and this creates an unbalanced digestive environment—and burning and pain are the result.

You might be astonished to learn that formal treatment of acid reflux—neutralizing excess stomach acid—has been around for about 200 years! Magnesium hydroxide was the active compound in this early treatment, and one of the first products available was Phillip's Milk of Magnesia®. Another acid neutralizer was developed nearly 100 years ago that uses calcium carbonate to neutralize excess acid, and was first available as Tums®.

Where does all of this excess acid come from? And why does it keep coming back? These are two questions to which everyone suffering from acid reflux always wants answers. Normally, when we eat, the cells in the lining of the stomach release a measured amount of hydrochloric acid into the stomach cavity to start the initial digestion process. The stomach protects itself from being damaged by the acid with a protective mucous coating that it secretes. But when too much acid is secreted into the stomach, the protective lining isn't enough, and the stomach can be damaged. Some of the excess acid can also percolate up into the esophagus, which has no protective mucous coating and can be easily injured. That's where the feeling of pain, that we call heartburn, comes from. One simple solution for treatment is the use of compounds containing magnesium hydroxide, calcium carbonate, and aluminum hydroxide. The excess acid in the stomach is neutralized by a simple chemical reaction, and pain subsides temporarily.

The down side to these compounds is that they are short acting and have some side effects. For example, ingesting too much magnesium causes diarrhea. Science has continued over the past 50 years to develop new ways to treat heartburn and indigestion. In the 1970s, a group of drugs, *histamine-2 blockers* (more commonly known in medicine as "histamine-2 antagonists"), were discovered and quickly found to be useful in reducing excess acid secretion by the stomach. This group of medications became the preferred means of treating heartburn, while the older antacids described above were used to supplement these drugs, as needed.

This was definitely a good start and improved treatment options, but the search continued for better and more effective ways to treat heartburn. This led to a big discovery in the 1980s of the *proton pump inhibitors*, a class of medications that slows the ability of the stomach's acid-secreting cells to release acid. This action essentially avoids the cascade of symptoms, since the root of the problem has been stopped: the extra acid release is directly blocked. It has proven so effective that proton pump inhibitors have become the mainstay of heartburn treatment when a simple antacid is not sufficient.

All three classes of antireflux medications—chemical antacids, histamine-2 blockers, and proton pump inhibitors—are currently used and widely available as over-the-counter treatments or by prescription. While you can easily purchase them without first having to see your doctor, if you have persistent heartburn, you should schedule a visit with your doctor to identify the optimal treatment strategy for you, and to rule out other disorders. As mentioned above, in some cases heartburn can actually be a symptom of heart disease.

## CLASSES OF ANTIREFLUX (ANTACID) MEDICATIONS

Chemical antacids:
- Aluminum hydroxide (Carafate®)
- Aluminum hydroxide plus magnesium carbonate (Gaviscon®, Gaviscon-2®)
- Calcium carbonate (Alka-Seltzer Heartburn Relief®, Tums®)
- Calcium carbonate plus magnesium hydroxide (Rolaids®)
- Magnesium hydroxide (Dulcolax Milk of Magnesia®, Phillips Milk of Magnesia®)

Histamine-2 blockers:
- Cimetidine (Tagamet®, Tagamet HB®)
- Famotidine (Pepcid®, Pepcid AC®)
- Nizatidine (Axid®, Axid AR®)
- Ranitidine (Zantac®)

Proton pump inhibitors:
- Dexlansoprazole (Dexilant®, Kapidex®)
- Esomeprazole (Nexium®)
- Lansoprazole (Prevacid®)
- Omeprazole (Prilosec®, Zegerid®)
- Pantoprazole (Protonix®)
- Rabeprazole (Aciphex®)

## Chemical Antacids

Many commonly used chemical antacids contain calcium carbonate to neutralize excess acid in the stomach (these include Tums and Alka-Seltzer Heartburn Relief). Others contain a combination of magnesium hydroxide and calcium carbonate (such as Rolaids) or a combination of magnesium carbonate and aluminum hydroxide (like Gaviscon) that acts to neutralize acid. It's easy to figure out which one you're taking—just read the ingredient label.

All chemical antacids are consumed *as needed* (when you feel heartburn). The instructions for appropriate use are listed on the package, including not only the suggested amount to take when you need them but also an amount *not to be exceeded in 24 hours*. Paying attention to this maximum amount is important, because significant side effects can occur when too much is consumed daily over a long period of time (weeks to months).

For all of these chemical antacids, you must be aware that, while they are very effective at neutralizing stomach acid and relieving your heartburn symptoms, they also *reduce the intestinal absorption of iron and folic acid* (a B vitamin, also known as folate). Both iron and folic acid are key to preventing anemia (as well as other diseases). Many people, especially premenopausal women, take extra iron daily to make sure there is enough to support normal blood cell function. Iron is needed for adequate production of red blood cells, which transport oxygen and nutrients throughout the body. If iron is low, and not enough red blood cells are created, the result is anemia.

Folic acid is also particularly important for women of child-bearing age, who are advised to take it before contemplating conception as well as throughout pregnancy to prevent developmental abnormalities of the nervous system. Importantly, if you are taking iron or folic acid supplements, *separate the ingestion of these supplements from the consumption of antacids by at least two hours.* Talk with your doctor to determine the optimal usage of both of these compounds.

## VITAMIN AND MINERAL RESTRICTIONS WHEN TAKING CHEMICAL ANTACIDS

- Do not take iron or folic acid supplements within two hours (before or after) of taking all chemical antacids.

- Do not consume foods or supplements containing vitamin C within two hours (before or after) of taking aluminum-containing antacids.

- Be mindful of total calcium intake when using calcium carbonate antacids. Determine total daily intake from all sources (foods, calcium supplements, and antacids) to stay below the safe upper limit for total calcium intake of 2,000 mg daily.

## Calcium Carbonate Antacids

For *calcium carbonate antacids*, the primary concern is consuming too much calcium on a daily basis. The most concentrated dietary source of calcium is dairy products, but a lot of calcium is also found in dark-green, leafy vegetables, with modest amounts found in grains and fruit. Calcium-fortified products (including some beverages and cereals) can contribute substantial amounts of calcium to the diet, along with multivitamin and mineral supplements as well as single-supplement forms of calcium. Calcium-containing antacids add to the total amount of calcium consumed daily.

American adults vary widely in their daily intake of calcium. The daily intake recommended by an expert group at the National Academy of Sciences is around 1,000 mg to maintain healthy bones. Americans fall both below and above this amount. The average American adult's calcium intake is around 600 to 800 mg daily. When it comes to calcium, more is not always better. A safe upper limit for daily calcium intake has been set at 2,500 mg daily for adults aged 19 to 50, and 2,000 mg daily for adults over age 50. If you go above this amount, over time you'll be at risk for developing kidney stones (very painful).

The important question is *How much calcium is in one of these antacids?* A standard calcium carbonate antacid tablet contains 500 mg of calcium carbonate. This is not 500 mg of calcium, but 200 mg (the carbonate part is 300 mg). Translated to the recommended amount to treat heartburn of two to four tablets each time you need it, this is a total of 400 to 800 mg of calcium. That's around one-half to three-quarters of your daily need, *before* you consume any foods. While the container may suggest that no more than 15 tablets should be ingested each day, that translates into a potentially health-damaging scenario for long-term calcium intake—about 3,000 mg of calcium (the safe upper limit is 2,000–2,500 mg).

> **SAFE UPPER LIMITS FOR DAILY INTAKE OF CALCIUM AND MAGNESIUM**
>
> **Calcium:** 2,000–2,500 mg total daily intake from all sources, including antacids (include calcium carbonate antacids to determine your total intake).
>
> **Magnesium:** 350 mg from antacids alone (include magnesium hydroxide and magnesium carbonate antacids to determine your intake). Daily intake from food is NOT included in this calculation.

The average American intake is 600–800 mg of calcium daily, so you would only need to take six to seven calcium carbonate tablets a day to reach the upper limit of safe ingestion (2,000 mg daily) if you are over age 50. If you're under age 50, it takes eight to nine tablets per day to reach the safe upper limit of intake (2,500 mg daily). Keep in mind that 600–800 mg is just the *average* daily intake of calcium for adult Americans, and many people—perhaps you too—are consuming much more.

Should you find that you regularly consume a large number of antacid tablets daily, which, when combined with your other dietary sources of calcium, exceeds the safe upper limit for calcium intake each day, it's important to pay a visit to your doctor to determine alternate treatments. You may need to control your heartburn with a different antacid, or perhaps a histamine-2 blocker, or a proton pump inhibitor.

---

If you choose to use calcium carbonate antacid tablets, it is important to pay attention to how many you consume every day to avoid ingesting too much calcium.

## *Magnesium Hydroxide and Magnesium Carbonate Antacids*

For *magnesium-containing antacids*, the concern is consuming too much magnesium, which can cause diarrhea. Besides the bathroom discomfort, chronic diarrhea can be a significant health problem because it can lead to serious water and salt imbalances in your body. If you use a magnesium-containing antacid, *the safe upper limit* of magnesium intake each day in the form of an *antacid* is about 350 mg to avoid diarrhea. (You also consume magnesium as a normal part of your diet, but the *safe upper limit* of intake is calculated by the National Academy of Sciences *in addition to* that normally present in the diet.)

A standard antacid containing magnesium hydroxide, such as regular strength Rolaids, contains 46 mg of magnesium per tablet, while extra-strength Gaviscon contains 44 mg of magnesium per tablet. For either of these products, this adds up to no more than about eight pills per day before side effects can be expected.

---

If you use magnesium-containing antacids, it is important to pay attention to how many you consume each day. If you find you're consuming too many on a regular basis, go see your doctor to discuss other treatment options for your heartburn.

---

## *Aluminum Hydroxide Antacids*

A third class of chemical antacids employs aluminum as an active ingredient to neutralize stomach acid. For this group, the aluminum hydroxide-containing antacids (including sucralfate [Carafate®]), the main issue is the absorption of small amounts of aluminum into the body. Almost all ingested aluminum is *not* absorbed and passes directly out of the body in bowel movements.

Although many issues have been raised about the potential negative health effects of aluminum over the years, *none* has proven to be a concern for normal, healthy people. The only clear medical situation of concern is advanced kidney (renal) disease, where the kidneys become less active in eliminating the small amounts of absorbed aluminum in the urine. Even so, it seems prudent to keep aluminum intake as low as possible to minimize even a potential risk. That's why it's important to monitor how many antacid tablets containing aluminum hydroxide you take each day.

You should also be aware that vitamin C (also known as ascorbic acid or ascorbate) greatly stimulates aluminum absorption by the intestines. To avoid any extra aluminum absorption, you should separate—by at least two hours—the ingestion of antacids containing aluminum hydroxide and food items containing vitamin C. Vitamin C is naturally found in citrus fruits and many citrus-containing beverages. It is also added to many beverages and other foods that don't normally contain it, along with vitamin and other dietary supplements. Even some cold remedies contain high levels of vitamin C.

If you take aluminum-containing antacids every day and the number regularly approaches or exceeds the maximum number specified on the container, you should discuss the issue with your doctor and identify a different treatment for your acid reflux, such as a histamine-2 blocker or a proton pump inhibitor.

## *Histamine-2 Blockers*

While the chemical antacids neutralize the acid already released into the stomach, a second group of medications was developed to slow acid release into the stomach as a way to reduce heartburn. This approach focuses on histamine, one of the signaling molecules in the stomach that controls acid-secreting cells. When histamine is released onto these cells, it binds to receptors on the cell surface and stimulates acid secretion. Don't get this action of histamine confused with that linked to allergic responses (such as hay fever). Histamine causes the effect in both situations, but different sets of cells are involved, and the effects are caused by histamine stimulating a different receptor found on the surface of each type of cell. The acid-secreting cells in the stomach have a "histamine-2" receptor, while the allergic response involves a "histamine-1" receptor.

Once the scientific discovery was made that histamine-2 receptors populated the surface of acid-secreting cells and caused acid secretion when tickled by histamine, drugs were quickly developed to *block* these sites to slow down how much acid would be produced. And blocking acid production proved to be quite effective in treating heartburn. Histamine-2 blockers remain a popular treatment option and are available in four different versions: cimetidine (Tagamet, Tagamet HB), famotidine (Pepcid®, Pepcid AC®), nizatidine (Axid®, Axid AR®), and ranitidine (Zantac®).

Like the chemical antacids, the histamine-2 blockers reduce stomach acidity and, as an indirect action, also reduce the intestinal absorption of iron and folic acid. So if you are taking an iron or folate supplement, separate its ingestion by at least two hours from the consumption of antacids.

**EATING GUIDELINES WHEN TAKING CIMETIDINE (TAGAMET, TAGAMET HB)**

- Limit alcohol, caffeine, nicotine intake
- Vitamin B12 supplementation may be needed (if cimetidine is used two or more years)
- Take with meals
- Do not take iron or folic acid supplements within two hours (before or after) of taking cimetidine

*Note:* The other histamine-2 blockers have only one of these guidelines: do not take iron or folic acid within 2 two hours (before or after) of taking any of the histamine-2 blockers.

Cimetidine should be ingested with food. The other histamine-2 blockers can be taken with or without food. Cimetidine slows the breakdown of alcohol, nicotine, and caffeine, so moderate your consumption of products containing them if you take cimetidine. The other blockers show only a negligible or very small effect. Because the long-term use of cimetidine (two or more years) has also been linked to reduced absorption of vitamin B12 and vitamin B12 deficiency, discuss this issue with your doctor and get your B12 level tested if you are using cimetidine consistently for more than a year. You may need to take a B12 supplement or select one of the other histamine-2 blockers.

Avoid taking *any* histamine-2 blocker at the same time as a chemical antacid. A chemical antacid can *slow* the absorption of the histamine-2 blocker, making it less effective in controlling stomach acid. If you are using medications in *both* of these antacid groups, take them two or more hours apart.

## *Proton Pump Inhibitors*

The proton pump inhibitors are the newest of the three classes of antacids. They are highly effective because they have the most direct action on acid-releasing cells. Proton pump inhibitors target the acid-secreting cells of the stomach and directly reduce their ability to secrete acid. This group of drugs directly blocks the actual acid-releasing mechanism of these cells. The following proton pump inhibitors are now used in the United States: omeprazole (Prilosec, Zegerid), esomeprazole (Nexium), lansoprazole (Prevacid), dexlansoprazole (Kapidex, Dexilant), pantoprazole (Protonix), and rabeprazole (Aciphex).

All drugs that decrease stomach acidity, no matter how they act, interfere with iron and folic acid absorption. This holds true for proton pump inhibitors, which reduce the intestinal absorption of iron and folic acid. If you are taking iron or folic acid supplements, separate supplement ingestion by at least two hours (before or after) from taking a proton pump inhibitor.

As for taking proton pump inhibitors with or without food, there are some differences among the members of this drug class: omeprazole (Prilosec, Zegerid), esomeprazole (Nexium) and lansoprazole (Prevacid) should be taken on an empty stomach because food reduces their absorption. The others—dexlansoprazole (Kapidex, Dexilant), pantoprazole (Protonix), and rabeprazole (Aciphex)—can be taken with or without food.

The only dietary supplement concerns are to avoid taking St. John's wort and ginkgo biloba with any of the proton pump inhibitors, as these herbal supplements cause the drugs to be metabolized more quickly. This results in making them less effective in controlling stomach acidity.

---

**DIETARY SUPPLEMENT ALERT!**

**Avoid with proton pump inhibitors:**

- St. John's wort
- Ginkgo biloba

---

There is also some evidence that the proton pump inhibitors decrease calcium absorption. If you're taking one of these drugs, it's good to make sure you consume at least the recommended daily allowance for calcium every day (about 1,000 mg daily). Using these drugs for extended periods of time (a year or more) can also lead to reduced vitamin B12 absorption and B12 deficiency, as well as hypomagnesemia (too little magnesium in the blood). The effect of the drugs on these vitamins and minerals can be corrected by using supplements.

## DIETARY CONCERNS WHEN TAKING PROTON PUMP INHIBITORS

Using daily for up to one year:
- Do not take iron or folic acid supplements within two hours (before or after) of taking a proton pump inhibitor.
- Take on an empty stomach: omeprazole (Prilosec, Zegerid), esomeprazole (Nexium), lansoprazole (Prevacid).
- Take with or without food: dexlansoprazole (Kapidex, Dexilant), pantoprazole (Protonix), rabeprazole (Aciphex).

Using daily for more than one year:
- Calcium—make sure to meet the daily requirement for calcium of 1,000 mg.
- Vitamin B12—supplements may be needed (your doctor can request a blood test to decide).
- Magnesium—supplements may be needed (your doctor can request a blood test to decide).

## PATIENT STORY: SUSAN

At age 39, Susan always felt she was in good health, and she'd often laugh and say jokingly, "I have an iron stomach, I can eat anything." So when she began having burning sensations in her chest after eating, she wondered if it was just a function of her age, or something else. Despite her demanding work schedule, she exercised daily and maintained a healthy diet. Susan first thought it could be her recent interest in spicy foods—she had become a big user of Sriracha and other hot sauces, but cutting out spicy foods made no substantial difference. She had read that caffeine could cause stomach acidity, and she swapped her morning coffee for herbal tea. But the burning persisted. It was apparent to Susan that she couldn't manage her problem with dietary changes alone, so she made an appointment with her doctor.

The initial medical recommendations were for Susan to lose a few pounds and take an over-the-counter medication as needed. Susan was nervous about taking any pills, but followed the recommendation of several friends who were taking Tums (including one who was taking it only as a source of calcium, not for heartburn). Susan also focused on losing weight and dropped 15 pounds in four months. She lost the weight by monitoring her food portions and eating more frequent meals. Her lifestyle changes paid off. The combination of her weight loss and choosing smaller, more frequent meals was a big boost. That alone reduced the frequency of her heartburn, and she found that Tums was very effective in neutralizing any excess stomach acid—and prevented any further discomfort. Susan was also pleased that she was using a calcium carbonate antacid because she was lactose intolerant and did not eat much dairy. She found this could double up as a calcium supplement to help meet her daily needs, which was great news.

## PATIENT STORY: HARRY

Harry had first started using Rolaids for his occasional heartburn while he was still in college. Now in his early 40s, he'd been using Gaviscon for the past few years with moderate success. But over the past few months he found he was taking it more often, yet still had heartburn, and noticed a new burning feeling further up, in his esophagus. While Gaviscon was helping with his symptoms, he was taking more pills and was worried he was approaching the upper recommended dose limit on most days. He also propped himself up on several pillows in bed at night, so he was not lying flat. His doctor had told him this might reduce any pain he might feel during the night, but sleeping on pillows made him uncomfortable and he slept poorly anyway. After discussing these chronic issues with his primary care doctor, Harry made an appointment with a gastroenterologist.

After an endoscopy (to determine the condition of his upper digestive track—esophagus, stomach, and the first part of the duodenum), the specialist recommended a proton pump inhibitor, and prescribed Nexium. Harry was glad to hear this would only require one daily dose, but he had to remember to take this on an empty stomach to promote correct and optimal absorption. He already took other medications for which consumption of food was not an issue, so he made a point of taking the Nexium at bedtime.

Over time, Harry became symptom-free and still enjoyed his favorite foods, but in more moderate portions. Harry definitely noticed that he remained symptom-free when he did not overeat. He learned to be more mindful, and even lost 10 pounds over about six months, which also helped reduce his heartburn.

# Chapter 6
# BLOOD PRESSURE (Antihypertensive) MEDICINES

Hypertension (high blood pressure) often begins as a silent risk. You don't feel that anything is wrong. Most likely, you first learn about it when your blood pressure is measured during a routine check-up at your doctor's office. And when your doctor finds it, he or she will immediately recommend you begin a medication and, as appropriate, lifestyle changes that, together, bring blood pressure back into the normal range.

Why are doctors so concerned about high blood pressure? Blood vessels are designed to withstand a good amount of pressure, but not an excessive amount. Too much pressure can rupture the blood vessels, with life-threatening consequences. For example, if high blood pressure causes blood vessels in the brain to break, the result can be a "hemorrhagic stroke," which involves the release of large volumes of blood into the brain under high pressure, which in turn can compress the brain and cause serious loss of brain function, some-times even death.

If blood pressure becomes elevated, the heart has to work harder to push blood into the circulation against the higher pressure. (For blood to flow out of the heart and into the blood vessels, the heart must generate an amount of pressure during contraction that is higher than that in the blood vessels.) Over a period of several years, the extra effort the heart must expend to pump blood at an above-normal pressure causes it to wear out more quickly, resulting in heart attack and heart failure at a relatively young age. For these and many other reasons, high blood pressure is treated to lower it as soon as it is discovered.

There are several types of drugs that are used to reduce high blood pressure. These drugs act on different parts of the cardiovascular system through mechanisms present in the body for controlling blood pressure. To understand how these drugs work, and why they are used, we need to know a little more about the organization of the heart and blood vessels that make up the cardiovascular system.

The cardiovascular system consists of the heart and two linked, but separate circulation loops. The heartbeat generates the pressure that moves blood through both loops. One loop is named the "pulmonary circulation," and cycles blood from the heart into the lungs (where it receives oxygen and gets rid of carbon dioxide) and then back to the heart. The second loop is the "systemic circulation," which cycles the freshly oxygenated blood to all other parts of the body (where oxygen is extracted from, and carbon dioxide inserted into the blood by the tissues). The blood then flows back to the heart, where it enters the pulmonary circulation, to begin the cycle anew. We need to focus a bit more on the systemic circulation to understand how blood pressure-lowering drugs work, since it is in this part of the circulation that hypertension almost always develops, when it occurs. And so it is here where the drugs act to lower blood pressure.

The heart pumps blood directly into the largest artery of the systemic circulation, the aorta, which then divides into the smaller arteries of each organ. These smaller arteries further subdivide into even smaller vessels in each organ called "arterioles," finally becoming the very tiny, thin vessels called "capillaries." It is in these tiniest of blood vessels—the capillaries—that nutrients, wastes, oxygen, and carbon dioxide are exchanged between the cells and the blood: the cells remove nourishing oxygen and nutrients from blood and replace them with carbon dioxide and other metabolic waste molecules. The capillaries then join into tiny veins called "venules," which join to form larger veins, and, further along, these larger veins join together in one very large vein (the vena cava), which finally arrives back at the heart.

Because of the physical design of the systemic circulation, the blood in the arteries is maintained at a much higher pressure than is found in the veins. It's the pressure in the arteries that is checked at your doctor's office. It is normal for the blood pressure to be higher in the arteries than in the veins—the systemic circulation is designed for it to be high. But arterial pressure can rise too high, for many reasons, and when it does, it becomes a health risk. But why would these arteries be under high pressure to begin with? It all comes down to the large arteries dividing up into tiny ones, to reach all the cells in the body. As the blood vessels get smaller, it gets harder to push the blood through them. Think of trying to expel water from your mouth through a large straw, as compared with a small, narrow one. You have to push much harder on the narrow one—creating higher pressure—to force the water through that smaller opening. The same is true with blood vessels: the heart (like your mouth in the example above) must generate high enough blood pressure to force blood to flow through the very narrow vessels.

The heart and arteries of the systemic circulation are designed to accommodate the higher pressure (compared with veins—the arteries are much thicker, and lined with muscle), but only within certain limits. That's where "knowing your numbers" is important. In a blood pressure reading (for example, 120/80), the top number, which is always higher than the lower number, measures the pressure in the arteries when the heart muscle contracts (beats). This is called the "systolic" pressure. The bottom number, the "diastolic" pressure, measures the pressure in the arteries when the heart muscle is resting between beats and refilling with blood.

A healthy arterial blood pressure is up to 120/80, and your body is designed to control blood pressure close to these values.

Surprisingly, the control of arterial blood pressure is a responsibility assigned to the brain, not the heart. The brain "measures" blood pressure through special pressure sensors in the arteries and can respond to increases in blood pressure in three different ways: it can slow down how fast blood enters the arteries from the heart. It can increase blood flow out of the arteries through the small vessels into the organs. And it can reduce the total blood volume—the amount of blood circulating in the entire cardiovascular system.

Any one of these responses can lower arterial pressure. The brain accomplishes these actions through nerves that run to the various parts of the cardiovascular system. It's a set of connections designed for your brain to make necessary, automatic corrections to blood pressure as you experience those stresses and strains of daily life. And when the system is not functioning normally and pressure rises too high, medications can help support a return into the normal pressure range. Because of the multiple ways that blood pressure can be lowered, there is a very large number of medications that can be effective. Often a combination of medications is used.

## *What Blood Pressure Numbers Mean to Your Health*

Arterial blood pressure can rise for many reasons. And none of them is good news for your health. If your blood pressure rises to 140/90 or higher, there is always the concern that this higher pressure might eventually cause blood vessels to burst. If this happens in the brain, as noted above, it is called a *stroke* and is often fatal. If your doctor finds that your blood pressure is above the normal range, he or she will probably prescribe a drug to take daily that reduces arterial blood pressure. Generally speaking, such "antihypertensive" drugs usually focus on reducing blood pressure in the arteries, because pressure is much higher in arteries than in veins, and for this reason is usually the cause of any health problems that develop.

## TABLE 2. KNOW YOUR NUMBERS: WHAT YOUR BLOOD PRESSURE READINGS MEAN

*Note:* Only your doctor can determine the specific health risks related to your blood pressure. Factors such as age and other diseases (like diabetes, kidney disease and obesity) can affect treatment.

| Blood Pressure Reading | Category | Action |
|---|---|---|
| 120/80 and lower | Normal | Maintain/ start healthy lifestyle habits* |
| Up to 139/89 | Pre-hypertension | Maintain/start healthy lifestyle habits |
| Between 140/90 and 159/99 | Stage 1 hypertension | Maintain/start healthy lifestyle habits; talk to your doctor about medication options |
| 160/100 and higher | Stage 2 hypertension | Maintain/start healthy lifestyle habits; talk to your doctor about medication options |

*A "healthy lifestyle" includes eating abundant fruits and vegetables, fiber-rich starches, and lean proteins; regular physical activity (a minimum of a 30-minute daily walk); stress management; and adequate sleep. Smoking cessation and weight loss are also important lifestyle factors that can help improve high blood pressure, along with medications.

## How Blood Pressure Medications Work

There are many mechanisms your body normally uses to moderate blood pressure, as discussed above. Drugs are designed to influence these mechanisms in a manner that lowers blood pressure. Some drugs relax the muscle lining the walls of the large arteries, which increases their size (diameter) and causes blood pressure to fall. Other drugs relax the muscles in the walls of *only* the tiny arterioles, which allows blood to flow *faster* out of the big arteries, reducing the amount of blood in these large arteries, which translates into reduced blood pressure. Another category of drugs slows down the flow of blood *out* of the heart into the arteries, which also results in lowering the volume of blood in the arteries and thereby arterial pressure. A variety of other drugs act to reduce the total volume of blood in the *entire* cardiovascular system, also causing arterial blood pressure to fall. All medications that are currently used to control high blood pressure are derived from this knowledge of how arterial blood pressure is controlled in the body.

In the simplest terms, drugs that reduce how fast the heart pumps blood into the arteries fall into two categories: *beta blockers* and *calcium channel blockers.* The beta blockers act indirectly on the heart by blocking nerve signals from the brain that are telling the heart to beat faster and stronger. The calcium channel blockers act on the heart muscle directly to turn down its pumping action. As a result, both types of drugs dial down the pumping action of the heart, and as a result lower blood pressure.

The alpha-1 blockers prevent nerve signals originating in the brain from signaling muscles in the artery walls, which normally causes them to contract. This results in a larger diameter (volume) of arteries (both big and small) in the body, resulting in a reduction in blood pressure.

Certain drugs act directly in the brain, causing it to turn down almost all nerve activity to the heart and blood vessels. These drugs, sometimes called "alpha-2 stimulators," either directly or indirectly stimulate alpha-2 receptors (specialized signaling sites on neurons in the brain) on brain neurons that control blood pressure.

Finally, there are many drugs that act through the kidneys to reduce blood volume (lowering blood volume in the circulation lowers blood pressure). One group is focused on a signal cascade that begins with nerves from the brain stimulating the release of a molecule (renin) by special kidney cells. This ultimately causes the release of a hormone (aldosterone) that controls urine volume. The cascade of actions is termed the renin-angiotensin-aldosterone system, and the drugs in this category interact with different components of this cascade to turn it down.

There are four medication groups that affect this system: angiotensin 2 blockers, Angiotensin-Converting Enzyme (ACE) inhibitors, direct renin inhibitors, and aldosterone blockers. Regardless of how this system is turned down, an increase in urine production occurs, which then lowers blood volume and pressure. Another group bypasses this cascade altogether and simply acts directly on urine-producing cells in the kidneys to boost urine formation. These are called "diuretics."

## TYPES OF MEDICATIONS THAT LOWER BLOOD PRESSURE (ANTIHYPERTENSIVES)

Beta blockers (beta-1 blockers):
- Atenolol (Tenormin®)
- Bisoprolol (Zebeta®)
- Metoprolol (Lopressor®, Toprol XL®)
- Nebivolol (Bystolic®)
- Acebutolol (Sectral®)

Beta blockers (nonselective):
- Nadolol (Corgard®)
- Propranolol (Hemangeol® [liquid], Inderal XA®, Inderal XL®, InnoPran XL®, Propranolol [tablet])

Calcium channel blockers:
- Amlodipine (Norvasc®)
- Felodipine (Plendil®)
- Nifedipine (Adalat®, Adalat CC®, Procardia®, Procardia XL®, Nifedipine ER®, Nifediac CC®, Nifedical XL®)
- Nisoldipine (Sular SR®)
- Diltiazem (Cardizem® [LA, CD], Cartia XT®, Dilacor XR®, Dilt® [CD, XR], Diltiazem CD®, Matzim LA®, Tiazac®, Taztia XT®)
- Verapamil (Calan®, Calan SR®, Covera-HS®, Isoptin SR®, Verelan® [SR, PM])

Alpha-1 blockers:
- Prazosin (Minipress®)
- Terazosin (Hytrin®)
- Silodosin (Rapaflo®)
- Alfuzosin (Uroxatral®)
- Tamsulosin (Flomax®)
- Doxazosin (Cardura®, Cardura XL®)
- Labetalol (Trandate® [dual function: also a beta-blocker])

Alpha-2 stimulators:
- Clonidine (Catapres®)
- Guanfacine (Tenex®)
- Methyldopa (Aldomet®)

ACE inhibitors:
- Benazepril (Lotensin®)
- Captopril (Capoten®)
- Enalapril (Vasotec®)
- Fosinopril (Monopril®)
- Lisinopril (Prinivil®, Zestril®)
- Moexipril (Univasc®)
- Perindopril (Aceon®)
- Quinapril (Accupril®)
- Ramipril (Altace®)
- Trandolapril (Mavik®)

Angiotensin 2 blockers:
- Azilsartin (Edarbi®)
- Candesartan (Atacand®)
- Eprosartan (Teveten®)
- Irbesartan (Avapro®)

- Losartan (Cozaar®)
- Olmesartan (Benicar®)
- Telmisartan (Micardis®)
- Valsartan (Diovan®)

Aldosterone blockers:
- Eplerenone (Inspra®)
- Spironolactone (Aldactone®)

Direct renin inhibitors:
- Aliskiren (Tekturna®)

Diuretics:
- Bumetanide (Burnex®)
- Furosemide (Lasix®)
- Ethacrynic acid (Edecrin®)
- Hydrochlorothiazide (Microzide®)
- Indapamide (Lozol®)
- Torsemide (Demadex®)
- Triamterene (Dyrenium®)

Since there are many ways blood pressure is regulated by the body, it's no surprise that there are many medications used to treat high blood pressure. To keep things clear and easy to understand, we're going to tackle each drug class—and medications within each one—separately when it comes to food and dietary supplements that might affect their action.

*As you read these sections, look for your own medication for specific recommendations of food and supplement interactions, as well as advice on taking them with or without food.*

While our discussion covers each drug separately, we're not assuming that you are taking just one drug to lower your blood pressure. In fact, your doctor may give you more than one to treat your high blood pressure most effectively. When taking multiple medications to control your blood pressure, it becomes *especially* important to discuss with your doctor the foods and dietary supplements you are taking. There is no standard answer: some foods and supplements can interfere with a drug's ability to lower blood pressure, while some can enhance the activity. This issue can become more complicated when you are taking more than one drug.

## *Blood Pressure Drug Interactions with Foods and Dietary Supplements*

Some foods that you eat, as well as alcohol and many dietary supplements, can *directly* raise or lower blood pressure on their own. They can also act *indirectly* to influence the ability of blood pressure drugs you are taking to lower blood pressure. This is important for you to know, especially if you are taking more than one antihypertensive drug.

### ALCOHOL AND BLOOD PRESSURE MEDICINES

Avoid or strictly limit intake of alcohol because it can
- Lower blood pressure
- Enhance the blood pressure lowering effects of your medication
- Lead to dizziness or fainting
- Increase sleepiness caused by some medications

### Dietary Supplements

Let's take a closer look at supplements. If you take a dietary supplement that by itself *lowers* blood pressure, it may enhance the blood pressure-lowering action of the drug you are taking. This added action means your blood pressure might fall too low, and you may get dizzy and pass out. If you take a supplement that *raises* blood pressure, it may reduce the blood pressure-lowering

135

effect of the drug you are taking. As a result, you may have to take more of the medication to overcome the opposing action of the supplement. At a higher dose you may experience more of the unpleasant side effects associated with its use.

## Herbal Supplements

Many herbal supplements can influence blood pressure and should be avoided when taking medications to treat high blood pressure. These are sold either as individual supplements, or as an ingredient in supplement "mixes" targeted for a variety of symptoms. Read the labels carefully to make sure you know what you're consuming. Here are some examples: *Bitter oranges* (such as Seville oranges) naturally contain compounds that raise blood pressure and heart rate. *Coenzyme Q10* has been shown to reduce blood pressure. *Ma-huang* (*Ephedra sinica*) supplements, which naturally contain compounds that raise blood pressure and heart rate, have been outlawed in the United States because of the illness and death resulting from their cardiovascular effects. *Asian ginseng* (Panax ginseng) can also reduce blood pressure; this is *not* true of American ginseng. Guarana (*Paullinia cupana*), which contains caffeine, can raise both blood pressure and heart rate. *Natural licorice* (*Glycyrrhiza glabra*) increases blood pressure, while *melatonin* and *hibiscus* can lower blood pressure under some conditions. Hawthorn has been reported to raise and to lower blood pressure, illustrating that effects of an herbal supplement can be present, but unpredictable.

This is only a partial list of some of the most popular dietary supplements affecting blood pressure; there are many others that may have an effect. If a supplement you take is *not* on our list, you can look online to identify which dietary supplements you take are thought to have blood pressure effects. Websites such as WebMD (webmd.com), Drugs.com, and the National Institutes of Health (ods.od.nih.gov/factsheets/list-all/; nccih.nih. gov/health/herbsataglance.htm) are all reliable sources.

Alcohol consumption can either lower blood pressure *or* enhance the blood pressure-lowering effects of the medications you are taking. This can lead to dizziness and fainting. Alcohol can also enhance the sleepiness caused by some antihypertensive drugs.

---

### DIETARY SUPPLEMENTS ALERT!

**Avoid when taking antihypertensive medications:**

- Hibiscus
- Bitter orange (*such as Seville oranges*)
- Coenzyme Q10
- Ma huang (*Ephedra sinica*)
- Asian ginseng (Panax ginseng)
- Guarana (*Paullinia cupana*)
- Hawthorn
- Natural licorice (*Glycyrrhiza glabra*)
- Melatonin
- St. John's wort

---

If you use one or more of the dietary supplements listed in the previous dietary supplement alert, it is best to discontinue their use, or at least inform your doctor that you use them. Have an open discussion with your doctor about your alcohol use, so you can be advised about adjusting intake, if necessary, to be compatible with your medication.

In the next section, we will review the nutrients and dietary supplements that may affect how well your antihypertensive drug works, and also *when to take it* (with or without food). Often it is not a specific food that affects the action of the medication but just the presence or absence of food; these are digestion and absorption concerns. We're discussing each medication group separately, for ease of use and understanding. Look for your own medication in each category for specific guidelines of foods and supplements to avoid, and when to take it.

## *Drugs That Act Primarily on the Heart and Blood Vessels to Lower Blood Pressure*

### Beta Blockers

Beta blockers act primarily on the heart to reduce blood pressure. They cause the heart to beat less rapidly and with less strength, which slows the flow of blood into the arteries, which in turn reduces blood pressure. One group of beta blockers (beta-1 blockers) works only on the heart, and includes atenolol (Tenormin), bisoprolol (Zebeta), metoprolol (Lopressor, Toprol XL), and nebivolol (Bystolic). Acebutolol (Spectral) may also be included in this grouping.

Nebivolol, bisoprolol, and acebutolol can be taken with food or on an empty stomach; it doesn't matter. You should discontinue using St. John's wort if you take *bisoprolol*, because this herb increases the breakdown of the drug, thus reducing the drug's ability to lower your blood pressure.

Atenolol can be taken with or without food, but choose one way and stick with it. Consistency is important because ingesting the drug with food boosts atenolol's absorption from the intestines. By taking your drug the same way each day (either with or without food), you'll get the same amount of drug into your body each day and the same amount of blood pressure reduction. As long as you are consistent, your doctor can easily adjust the dose to get the desired drop in blood pressure. When you take atenolol with orange juice (*any* kind of orange juice), it reduces drug absorption from the intestines. *Don't drink orange juice within four hours (before or after) of taking the drug.* Atenolol absorption is also reduced if you take the medicine at the same time as a calcium supplement (included in multivitamins, some antacids, or calcium-fortified juices). Separate taking the drug and any calcium supplement by about four hours.

Metoprolol is available as either a standard tablet or in an extended-release pill (Toprol XL). The form makes a big difference in how the medication is absorbed into your body. For the standard tablet, absorption is increased when ingested with food, so take it consistently either with food or on an empty stomach. But because the extended-release pill is released gradually and absorbed slowly over the course of the entire day, it can be ingested without regard to time of food ingestion.

A second group of beta blockers is termed "nonselective" because they act on the heart to lower blood pressure but also block beta receptors elsewhere in the body. This group includes nadolol (Corgard) and propranolol (Hemangeol [liquid]; Inderal XA; Inderal XL; InnoPran XL; Propranolol [tablet]).

Nadolol can be taken either on an empty stomach or with food. Green tea blocks the intestinal absorption of nadolol and reduces its ability to lower blood pressure. *You should avoid drinking green tea if you take nadolol.*

Propranolol tablets should be taken on an empty stomach. The extended-release pills (XA and XL designations) can be taken with or without food but take them consistently one way or the other, since food affects drug absorption. When using the liquid form (Hemangeol), take the dose with or just after a meal because this formulation can cause hypoglycemia if ingested on an empty stomach.

If you use St. John's wort, you should stop taking this supplement because it will reduce the availability of propranolol within the body, decreasing its ability to lower blood pressure. Also avoid taking aluminum-containing antacids together with propranolol, as these antacids block propranolol absorption and reduce its effects. Take the drug at least three hours before or after using this group of antacids (or switch to a nonaluminum type).

## Calcium Channel Blockers

Calcium channel blockers provide a "dual action" to reduce blood pressure by acting both on the heart and on blood vessels. These drugs reduce how fast the heart pumps blood into the circulation. It also relaxes the blood vessels, causing them to open up wider. Together, these actions lower blood pressure. There is a wide variety of medications in this class: amlodipine (Norvasc), felodipine (Plendil), and nifedipine (Adalat, Adalat CC, Procardia, Procardia XL, Nifedipine ER, Nifediac CC, Nifedical XL). Others are nisoldipine (Sular SR), diltiazem (Cardizem [LA, CD], Cartia XT, Dilacor XR, Dilt [CD, XR], Diltiazem CD, Matzim LA, Tiazac, Taztia XT), and verapamil (Calan, Calan SR, Covera-HS, Isoptin SR, Verelan® [SR, PM]).

For all of the calcium channel blockers, you should monitor calcium-containing products (for example, calcium-fortified juices, calcium supplements, calcium-containing multivitamins, calcium-containing antacids) unless advised differently by your doctor. *Do not exceed a daily total intake of calcium of around 1,000 mg daily, from all sources, including food.* And check with your doctor if you take individual vitamin D supplements that are higher than the recommended daily intake of 400–800 IU (international units), because vitamin D enhances calcium absorption from the intestine (indirectly boosting calcium intake). Calcium channel blockers reduce blood pressure by slowing the uptake of calcium into the cells of the heart and blood vessels. Elevated blood calcium levels due to high intake from the diet can reduce the ability of the drug to block cellular calcium uptake, and thus its ability to lower blood pressure.

You should not use St. John's wort, as the herbal supplement increases the breakdown of these drugs in the body, so your medication dosage will be less effective in reducing your blood pressure. If you eat more than half a grapefruit or more than a small glass of grapefruit juice (6–8 oz) each day, you should reduce your intake of these products or eliminate them from your diet (check with your doctor). Grapefruit slows the breakdown of the drug, and your blood pressure may fall too low, resulting in dizziness or faintness.

**FOODS AND SUPPLEMENTS TO LIMIT WHEN TAKING CALCIUM CHANNEL BLOCKERS**

- Grapefruit and grapefruit juice

- Calcium-fortified foods (such as orange juice)

- Calcium-containing antacids

- Calcium supplements

- St. John's wort

- Melatonin (eliminate if taking amlodipine, felodipine, nifedipine, nisoldipine)

- Red yeast rice (eliminate when taking verapamil or diltiazem, if also taking a statin drug)

There are some additional guidelines for only certain calcium channel blocker medications. If you specifically take amlodipine, felodipine, nifedipine or nisoldipine, do *not* take melatonin because it can reduce the effectiveness of the drug in lowering blood pressure. (It is not yet known if this is also true for other calcium channel blockers.)

And if you take either verapamil or diltiazem and eat red yeast rice, which naturally contains lovastatin, you should be aware that there is a direct connection between lovastatin and these two blood pressure-lowering medicines. Verapamil and diltiazem block the breakdown of lovastatin in the body, and blood levels will be higher as a result. *There is no harm if you eat red yeast rice, as long as you are not also taking lovastatin as a medication to lower high cholesterol levels.* If you are taking lovastatin as a drug (Mevacor®) and eating red yeast rice, and are also placed on verapamil or diltiazem to lower blood pressure, you may inadvertently cause blood lovastatin levels to rise high enough to enhance the unpleasant side effects of lovastatin (such as muscle pain and damage). This is an example of a combination of drugs and supplements leading to surprising and unpleasant effects. Discuss this issue with your doctor, if it applies to you.

Should you take a calcium channel blocker with food, or on any empty stomach? Calcium channel blockers can differ in this regard. You should carefully read the instructions provided to you by your pharmacist, or ask for this information when you pick up your prescription. The advice varies depending on your specific medication, but here is a brief summary:

Amlodipine and felodipine can be taken with food or on an empty stomach. But if you take felodipine with food, take it with a light meal, up to around 250 calories.

(A large meal greatly increases felodipine absorption, and too much medication can get into your body.)

Nisoldipine should be taken a few hours before or after a meal. Do not take this medicine with food because absorption is affected.

Nifedipine tablets can be taken with food or on an empty stomach. However, there are several extended-release forms of nifedipine, and they differ regarding whether they should be taken with food or not. Make sure you read the instructions provided by your pharmacist carefully, and ask your pharmacist or doctor if you are not entirely sure.

Diltiazem tablets should be taken before meals and at bedtime. However, the various extended-release pills differ in their dietary instructions. If you are taking an extended-release pill, read the instructions carefully, or check with your pharmacist or doctor for clarification about combining your medication with foods.

Most forms of verapamil can be taken with or without food. However, Calan SR and Isoptin SR should be taken with food.

## Alpha-1 Blockers

Alpha-1 blockers reduce blood pressure primarily by relaxing the muscle layer lining the walls of large and small blood vessels. When these muscles relax, the blood vessels open up and become wider. This larger opening itself reduces blood pressure; plus, the blood flows more easily through the smaller vessels—further helping to reduce pressure.

The alpha-1 blockers currently in use in the United States are prazosin (Minipress), terazosin (Hytrin), silodosin (Rapaflo), alfuzosin (Uroxatral), tamsulosin (Flomax), and doxazosin (Cardura, Cardura XL). One additional drug, labetalol (Trandate), is both an alpha-1 blocker and a beta blocker. (In addition to their use in controlling blood pressure, alpha-1 blockers are also used to treat benign prostatic hypertrophy.)

If you take alfuzosin, doxazosin, silodosin, or tamsulosin, you should *not* use St. John's wort. This herbal supplement increases the breakdown of these drugs in the body, making them less effective in reducing blood pressure. As a result, your blood pressure may continue to be too high. If you eat more than half a grapefruit or more than a small glass of grapefruit juice (6–8 oz) each day, you should reduce your intake of these products or eliminate them from your diet (check with your doctor). Ingesting grapefruit slows the breakdown of alfuzosin, silodosin, and tamsulosin, and your blood pressure may fall too far. As a result, you may become dizzy or faint.

When it comes to "food or no food" with these medicines, read the package insert or check with your pharmacist or doctor, because the advice varies with each medication. Doxazosin, prazosin, and terazosin can be taken either on an empty stomach or with food. Cardura XL (the extended-release form of doxazosin) should be taken with the morning meal each day. Silodosin and labetalol should be taken along with food. Alfuzosin should be taken with a meal at the same time each day, while tamsulosin should be taken 30 minutes after a meal at the same time each day.

## Alpha-2 Stimulators

Alpha-2 stimulators lower blood pressure by acting in the brain. These medications turn down the flow of nerve signals from the brain to the heart and blood vessels that normally cause blood pressure to rise. These nerves normally act to increase the pumping of blood by the heart, and the constriction of the arteries; slowing down these signals slows the pumping action of the heart and widens the arteries, which are effective ways to lower blood pressure. The alpha-2 stimulators currently used in the United States are clonidine (Catapres), guanfacine (Tenex) and methyldopa (Aldomet).

All alpha-2 stimulators can make you feel sleepy. If you take any of these drugs, avoid alcohol and herbal supplements such as kava and valerian. When consumed with these medications, they can make you even sleepier.

Only guanfacine has specific foods and herbal supplements to avoid. If you take this medicine, limit your daily ingestion of grapefruit products—no more than half a grapefruit or a small glass of grapefruit juice (6–8 oz). Ingesting grapefruit *slows* this drug's breakdown, so more stays in your body, as if the dose were higher. Your blood pressure may then fall too far, and you may feel dizzy or faint. You should not use St. John's wort with guanfacine because it increases the breakdown of the medication in the body. This makes the medication *less* effective in reducing blood pressure, and your pressure may continue to be too high.

For methyldopa, if you take an iron supplement (for example, a multivitamin with iron), take it at least two hours before or after you take methyldopa. Iron reduces the absorption and effectiveness of this drug, so your prescribed dose might not lower your pressure adequately.

When it comes to taking these drugs with or without food, it's important to follow these guidelines to make sure you're getting the correct intended dose. Clonidine, guanfacine, and methyldopa can be taken on an empty stomach or with food. However, remember, *do not take methyldopa with meals containing large amounts of protein* because, if you do, the availability of methyldopa to the brain may be reduced, making the drug less effective in lowering blood pressure.

# Drugs with Actions Primarily on the Kidneys

Another way to lower blood pressure is to increase urine production, which lowers the overall amount of blood circulating in the body (blood volume). These medications modify the elimination of several very important body electrolytes (salts, such as sodium and potassium). If you take one or more of these drugs, it is *very* important to pay attention to blood levels and dietary intake of these electrolytes. Dietary changes can influence the blood levels of sodium and potassium in your blood. Depending on your medication and the dose, you may need to take a supplement, increase your dietary intake, or have a more controlled diet to limit your intake of these compounds. Discuss these dietary issues with your doctor and, if needed, schedule an appointment with a registered dietician for specific food and menu recommendations.

## Angiotensin-Converting Enzyme Inhibitors

Angiotensin-Converting Enzyme (ACE) inhibitors prevent the formation of a compound, angiotensin 2, that raises blood pressure through direct action on arteries and indirect action on the kidneys. Angiotensin 2 directly constricts blood vessels (arteries), causing their diameters to become smaller, which itself raises blood pressure. Angiotensin 2 also stimulates the production of a hormone, aldosterone, which reduces the production of urine by the kidneys, thus causing water to be retained by the body. The result is that the total volume of blood in the cardiovascular system increases, which raises blood pressure. When these actions are blocked by an ACE inhibitor (by preventing the formation of angiotensin 2), blood pressure drops. That's how ACE inhibitors work.

Important to keep in mind here, in relation to food and dietary supplements, is how aldosterone reduces water loss through the formation of urine by the kidneys. Aldosterone prevents water loss in the kidneys by preventing salt (sodium) loss. The explanation of why water loss is tied to sodium loss is beyond the scope of this book. Suffice it to say that, if the kidneys retain sodium, they retain water; if they let sodium go out in the urine, water goes along too. Aldosterone causes the kidneys to retain sodium and, thus, water, too. It follows that, if an ACE inhibitor causes less aldosterone to be produced, it has the effect of causing sodium to be lost from the body, along with water. A related, important fact is that aldosterone also causes an increase in the removal of potassium in the urine, for reasons we won't go into here. The ACE inhibitor, by blocking aldosterone formation, leads to potassium being retained by the body and an increase in blood potassium levels.

The effect of ACE inhibitors in causing potassium to be retained and blood potassium levels to rise is medically important. If blood potassium rises too much, an irregular heartbeat can develop, which sometimes leads to a heart attack. For this reason, if you are taking an ACE inhibitor, your doctor will monitor electrolyte levels in your blood to make sure they are in the normal range. This includes potassium. If the blood potassium level is above normal, you can help to reduce it by taking stock of the sources of potassium in your diet and then reducing your intake of items containing this electrolyte. Indeed, your doctor may ask you to limit dietary potassium intake—including your intake of potassium-rich foods, such as dark-green, leafy vegetables (spinach, cabbage, and kale), and vine-based plants (tomatoes, cucumbers, zucchini, and eggplant). Consult with a registered dietician for further personalized dietary advice.

The potassium issue is sufficiently important that the FDA recommends that patients taking ACE inhibitors *not* use the following compounds without consulting their doctor: potassium-sparing diuretics, potassium supplements, or potassium-containing salt substitutes. *You may not realize that some salt substitutes contain potassium. If you are using a salt substitute, check the label for potassium and, if present, find another product that does not contain potassium.*

The ACE inhibitors presently available in the United States are benazepril (Lotensin), captopril (Capoten), enalapril (Vasotec), fosinopril (Monopril), Lisinopril (Prinivil, Zestril), moexipril (Univasc), perindopril (Aceon), quinapril (Accupril), ramipril (Altace), and trandolapril (Mavik).

In addition to potassium, there is one other item that you may include in your diet that opposes the action of the ACE inhibitors: natural licorice. Natural licorice has an action on the kidneys that mimics the action of aldosterone. It therefore opposes one of the main actions of the ACE inhibitor, which is to reduce aldosterone. If you love natural licorice, or use it as an herbal supplement, and regularly consume 3 ounces or more, you should stop while taking an ACE inhibitor. It may diminish the blood pressure-lowering effect of the drug.

Aside from potassium and natural licorice, the different medications in this group of drugs vary in food and supplement interactions. Look for your specific drug in this section and check with your pharmacist or doctor for further clarification.

*Captopril, fosinopril, lisinopril, and quinapril should not be taken with antacids or supplements containing magnesium or aluminum.* When you take antacids or such supplements at the same time as these medications, you can *reduce* their absorption and decrease their effectiveness in lowering blood pressure.

Captopril, moexipril, perindopril, and quinapril should be taken an hour or two before a meal, because food can reduce their absorption and their ability to lower blood pressure. All other drugs in this class can be taken without regard to food.

Captopril should *not* be taken with iron supplements. Iron binds to captopril in the intestines, reducing its absorption into the blood. Tell your doctor if you are taking an iron supplement, as you may be given a different drug in this class (only captopril has this effect). Another possible option is to separate taking captopril from your iron supplement by at least two hours. Also, keep in mind that long-term use of captopril can lead to zinc deficiency. If you are taking captopril, and develop signs of zinc deficiency (from a blood test), your doctor may have you take a different drug of the same class. While a zinc supplement is an option, it is unlikely that this would be recommended; switching to another drug in this class is simpler.

## LIMIT POTASSIUM WITH BLOOD PRESSURE MEDICINES AFFECTING KIDNEY FUNCTION

For all medications *except* diuretics avoid or limit the following potassium sources:
- Potassium-containing salt substitutes
- Potassium supplements
- Potassium-rich foods (dark-green, leafy vegetables; vine-based plants like tomatoes)

## Angiotensin 2 Blockers

Angiotensin 2 blockers (antagonists) act in a very similar manner to the ACE inhibitors: they block the biological actions of angiotensin 2. Angiotensin 2 naturally constricts blood vessels and stimulates the production of aldosterone, which reduces urine production in the kidneys. The effect of these actions is to raise blood pressure. By blocking these actions of angiotensin 2, this group of drugs lowers blood pressure.

The angiotensin 2 blockers in use in the United States are azilsartin (Edarbi), candesartan (Atacand), eprosartan (Teveten), irbesartan (Avapro), losartan (Cozaar), olmesartan (Benicar), telmisartan (Micardis), and valsartan (Diovan).

All angiotensin 2 blockers, like the ACE inhibitors described earlier, can cause the kidneys to retain potassium. Abnormally high potassium levels in the blood can cause the heart to malfunction, so it's important to avoid consuming potassium-containing salt substitutes, potassium supplements, and foods that are especially rich in potassium.

The effects of all angiotensin 2 blockers to reduce aldosterone production and actions on the kidneys are opposed by natural licorice, which mimics the action of aldosterone. Therefore, as with the ACE inhibitors, if you regularly consume 3 or more ounces of natural licorice, you should stop while taking an angiotensin 2 blocker, as the licorice may reduce the blood pressure-lowering effect of the drug.

Only losartan (Cozaar) has specific food and supplement restrictions. If you ingest grapefruit, grapefruit juice, pomelo, or Seville oranges, you should limit your intake of these fruits, because their ingestion may reduce the effects of losartan. You should also avoid taking St. John's wort with this medication, because it, too, will reduce the effectiveness of the drug in lowering blood pressure.

With one exception—valsartan (Diovan)—all of these drugs can be taken without regard to food. Valsartan must be taken consistently, either always with food, or always on an empty stomach. Food slows the absorption of this drug into the blood and can reduce the blood pressure-lowering effect. If you take the drug consistently with or without food, your doctor can monitor its effect and adjust your dose to reach the desired reduction in blood pressure.

## Aldosterone Blockers

Aldosterone blockers directly block the actions of aldosterone on the kidneys. There are currently two drugs in this class of antihypertensive agents: eplerenone (Inspra) and spironolactone (Aldactone). When aldosterone is doing its job, urine volume is low. By preventing this action, these drugs cause a larger amount of urine to form and be excreted. This effect reduces blood volume (because there is less water in the body) and lowers blood pressure.

For both of these drugs, you might experience elevated potassium levels in your blood, This can cause irregular heartbeat, so you should be careful about how much potassium you consume in your diet each day. Avoid potassium-containing salt substitutes and potassium supplements, and limit your intake of vegetables containing high amounts of potassium (such as dark-green, leafy vegetables and vine-based plants, including tomatoes, zucchini, cucumbers, and eggplant). For this group of drugs, you do *not* need to avoid licorice, since the drugs block the aldosterone receptor, which licorice is thought to need to cause its aldosterone-like effects.

When taking eplerenone (Inspra), restrict your intake of grapefruit, bitter oranges (such as Seville), and pomelo, whether in whole fruit or as a juice. Limit grapefruit to no more than one-half in a day or 6–8 ounces of grapefruit juice daily. Eating these fruits slows the body's ability to break down this drug, causing a larger reduction in blood pressure than expected. As a result, you may feel dizzy, faint, or experience some of the other side effects of this drug. You can take eplerenone (Inspra) alone or with food, it doesn't matter.

Avoid St. John's wort if you take eplerenone. Consumption of this herb may speed up its breakdown in your body, which may result in a reduced effect on lowering your blood pressure.

If your doctor prescribes spironolactone (Aldactone), the only diet-related issue is to take it with food to ensure it is maximally absorbed. Neither grapefruit juice nor St. John's wort alters the action of this drug.

### Direct Renin Inhibitors

Only one direct renin inhibitor is in use in the United States: aliskiren (Tekturna). This drug indirectly blocks the formation and action of aldosterone in the kidneys, which leads to a greater urine volume. When urine volume increases, blood pressure drops. As with other drugs in this class that act on the kidney to lower blood pressure, potassium levels in the blood could be elevated. Your doctor will monitor your blood potassium level, to ensure it remains in the normal range. This is important, because elevated potassium levels can lead to irregular heartbeat.

You must be careful about how much potassium you consume in your diet each day. Avoid potassium-containing salt substitutes and potassium supplements, and limit your intake of vegetables that contain high amounts of potassium (such as dark-green, leafy vegetables and vine-based plants, such as tomatoes, zucchini, cucumbers, and eggplant).

The absorption of aliskiren is also *slowed* by the ingestion of apple, orange, and grapefruit juice. This may make the drug *less* effective, and your blood pressure may remain too high. Avoid these fruits and juices if you take this medication.

The effects of aliskiren to reduce aldosterone production and actions on the kidneys are opposed by natural licorice. Therefore, as with ACE inhibitors and angiotensin 2 blockers, if you regularly consume 3 or more ounces of natural licorice, stop while taking aliskiren, as licorice may reduce the blood pressure-lowering effect of the drug.

When it comes to meals, foods containing fat slow the absorption of aliskiren into the blood. Remember to take the drug consistently one way or the other: either always with food or always on an empty stomach. Your doctor can adjust the amount of drug you take to allow for your dietary preference for fat. If you decide to change the composition of your diet, inform your doctor, so that your dose can be adjusted, if necessary.

## Diuretics

Diuretics act *directly* on the kidney to modify salt and water balance. Like all the other medicines that affect kidney function, diuretics cause urine output to increase, which results in lower blood pressure. Diuretics (nicknamed "water pills" by many users) also increase the elimination of electrolytes, including sodium, potassium, chloride and magnesium. Some diuretics also affect calcium elimination.

These drugs increase sodium elimination in the urine, which causes the increase in urine volume, which in turn lowers blood volume and thus blood pressure. But each of these drugs acts slightly differently on the basis of which electrolytes they affect, such as sodium, potassium, magnesium, calcium, or a combination of these; knowing these differences is important. When it comes to making dietary changes to avoid having too much or too little of these electrolytes in your body as a result of taking a diuretic, knowledge is power. Foods definitely can influence your nutritional status when taking diuretics.

Bumetanide (Burnex), furosemide (Lasix), ethacrynic acid (Edecrin) and torsemide (Demadex) make up one group of diuretics called "loop diuretics." These drugs *increase* sodium, chlorine, potassium, magnesium, and calcium loss in the urine. It is possible that blood levels of one or more of these elements may fall as a consequence, so your doctor will probably monitor your blood levels of these elements to make sure they are in the normal range of values. If they are low, your doctor may ask you to take an appropriate supplement or to eat more of certain foods to restore blood levels to normal. *It's important to take these medicines on an empty stomach.* Food reduces their absorption and will reduce their blood pressure-lowering effect.

A second group of diuretics is called "thiazide diuretics." This group includes hydrochlorothiazide (Microzide) and indapamide (Lozol). These diuretics can be taken *with* food. Food does *not* affect their absorption. Like the loop diuretics above, the thiazide diuretics promote urine production by increasing sodium loss from the kidneys; a loss of potassium also occurs. Yet, calcium elimination may be reduced. These changes can result in levels of potassium that are too low, or calcium levels that are too high, in the bloodstream. That's why your doctor will regularly monitor these electrolytes in your blood. If your potassium level is too low, your doctor may advise a change in diet to include potassium-rich foods, or a potassium supplement. A reduction in calcium intake will likely be advised if the blood level becomes too high. Vitamin D stimulates calcium absorption from the intestines, so, if you take a vitamin D supplement, you may also be asked to reduce the amount you take.

Chronic use of hydrochlorothiazide (Microzide) can also increase magnesium loss in the urine, particularly in elderly individuals. If your blood level of magnesium has declined, you may be asked to add more of this element to your diet.

One medication accounts for a third type of diuretic drug: triamterene (Dyrenium). This diuretic differs from the others in that, it is *"potassium sparing."* Rather than causing potassium elimination in the urine, this drug actually reduces its excretion. It may be taken with or without food. Taking it with food usually minimizes the gastric upset that sometimes occurs.

The only potential dietary issue with this drug concerns potassium retention. If blood potassium levels rise above the normal range while you are taking this drug, your doctor will ask you to reduce the amount of potassium you ingest each day. If so, you should avoid potassium-containing salt substitutes, if you use them, as well as taking in potassium from other sources, including some multivitamin pills, other dietary supplements, and foods naturally high in potassium.

A modest reduction in the levels and action of folic acid can occur, particularly when used by people who are already folic acid deficient. An easy solution is to increase the ingestion of foods containing folic acid, or take a folic acid supplement. Folic acid deficiency causes a form of anemia and is also a concern during the first trimester of pregnancy, when it is particularly important in the early development of the fetus' nervous system. Your doctor will monitor your blood folate level and recommend an increase in intake, if necessary.

## PATIENT STORY: NANCY

Nancy had a family history of heart disease and high blood pressure. She had always followed a healthy lifestyle since her 20s. Nancy ate lots of fruits and vegetables, chicken and fish, and avoided most processed foods (and extra salt). She walked regularly for exercise—at least two to three miles daily. This helped her maintain a healthy and stable weight for the past 30 years.

Now at age 52, Nancy was at her yearly checkup when her blood pressure was measured at 150/100 millimeters of mercury (mmHg)—which scared her. Over the years, in past doctor visits, she'd have an occasional elevated reading but she'd chalk it up to nerves. Her doctor thought that her genetics contributed to this, and her healthy lifestyle was still a major health plus—particularly since her pressure was now in the hypertensive range.

Nancy agreed to start on a low dose of irbesartan (an angiotensin 2 blocker) of 75 mg daily (the lowest starting dose). Much to her delight, Nancy's pressure dropped to a normal range. Her doctor was very pleased with the outcome, and Nancy has stayed on this dose of Avapro for the past four years.

After monitoring her blood pressure at home as well, Nancy noticed that stress caused her pressure to bump up. She took a class in meditation, and, although she was not a believer at first, she found that the mind exercises she learned were a big help. She felt her response to stress was managed much better. Nancy's doctor believes that her healthy lifestyle, stable weight, and improved stress management all contribute to her maintaining a normal blood pressure on a low dose of medication.

## PATIENT STORY: GREG

At age 50, Greg had high blood pressure for several years. His primary care doctor had started him on medication (an alpha-1 blocker, terazosin [Hytrin]) about five years ago. With some family history of heart disease, and slowly rising blood pressure, Greg had an open discussion with his doctor. To better support his health, Greg had some lifestyle changes to make. He agreed to work on losing 15 pounds of the weight he had gained over the past five years. He agreed with his doctor that this would improve his blood pressure, along with the medication. While the mutual goal was to use as few medications as possible, his doctor added a thiazide diuretic to his therapy to remove excess fluid from his body and provide a second way to lower his blood pressure.

Greg was warned by his doctor that diuretics can decrease his potassium, so he tried to include more potassium-rich foods in his diet to keep his levels from dropping. Unfortunately, when he returned to his doctor for regular blood work, he found his blood potassium level was low. He was surprised to hear that, but his doctor said that often a dietary change is not sufficient to offset the medication effects on potassium. He asked Greg to add a daily potassium supplement and redid his blood work after a few weeks. His numbers were now in the normal range—a definite plus for Greg. Greg embraced healthy eating, including a variety of fresh foods, in moderate portions. And he's slowly losing those extra pounds with smarter eating and a daily 30-minute walk—both of which contribute to healthy blood pressure. Greg is also working hard at other lifestyle changes that are under his control, with the hope that he will be limited to two medications to help keep his blood pressure in the normal range.

# Chapter 7
# CHOLESTEROL-LOWERING MEDICINES

## *Why We Need Cholesterol*

Cholesterol-lowering drugs are among the most widely used medications in the world. Your body produces cholesterol, and it's found in many foods. But what is it for? Clearly, there is a reason for cholesterol because your liver naturally makes it, but why? You may be surprised to know that your body *does* need cholesterol as a foundation of good health in many ways. For example, cholesterol is used by the body to make hormones that help your body respond to physical and mental stress. It also is the foundation for the production of sex hormones, contributing to regulation of body actions from puberty to pregnancy, including all aspects of reproductive function.

In fact, we cannot live without cholesterol, and that's why your liver is able to make it—just in case you don't get enough from the diet—which is a perfect example of the natural "checks and balances" in your body. Cholesterol is made in the liver, pumped out and transported by the bloodstream to all parts of the body. And while the liver is a major source of cholesterol for the body, what we eat also can be a big contributor to the total amount of cholesterol circulating in the bloodstream. Both cholesterol and saturated fat in the diet can boost blood cholesterol levels. And when it comes to total cholesterol in the body, too much can cause some major cardiovascular health risks. Excess levels of cholesterol can contribute to clogged blood vessels, often resulting in an increased risk of heart disease, heart attack, or stroke.

While the total *amount* of cholesterol in blood is a key reflection of how much your body tissues are exposed to, there are several types of cholesterol that contribute. There are two versions of cholesterol—one "good" and one "bad"—that are involved with transporting cholesterol throughout the body. The "good" form of cholesterol, high-density lipoprotein (HDL; think "H" for "healthy") helps to remove cholesterol deposits from the walls of blood vessels, keeping them clean and clog-free. You want this number to be high. The "bad" form of cholesterol, low-density lipoprotein (LDL; think "L" for "lousy") is the form of cholesterol that deposits cholesterol onto the blood vessel walls, where it sticks and has the potential to clog up the vessel. You want this number to be low.

Monitoring this "family" of cholesterols is important to good health. When your total cholesterol level is too high, and the balance between good and bad cholesterol is off, it's time to intervene. It's important to know your numbers—to keep your HDL high, and your LDL low, within a healthy range.

Scientific studies help determine the healthy range of blood cholesterol levels. Because blood cholesterol levels are often a strong predictor of future cardiovascular illness, it's important to understand where any rise in levels is coming from to determine the best treatment strategy. And cholesterol comes only from two places: foods and what the liver produces. When cholesterol levels are *higher* than the recommended range for good health, you must work to lower them.

The first line of treatment prescribed for elevated cholesterol is usually a change in the diet. That can definitely be a solution for some people, but it doesn't always work. Even with a dietary intervention to cut down on cholesterol and saturated fat consumed in the diet, it's often not enough. When dietary changes do not lower cholesterol levels to a healthy level, it means that the liver is producing too much for the body's needs. That's where medications can help.

## *Dietary Steps to Reduce Cholesterol*

A diet aiming to reduce cholesterol must be low in both cholesterol and saturated fat. Cholesterol and saturated fat overlap in a lot of foods (like fatty red meat), but sometimes they are separate (eggs and shrimp are cholesterol-rich but low in saturated fat). Both must be monitored to optimize the chance that a dietary intervention alone will lower cholesterol levels to a healthy range.

A six-month trial of a diet that is low in cholesterol and saturated fat can help define whether the major cause of elevated cholesterol is from eating too much cholesterol or from the body making too much, or even some combination of the two. The American Heart Association and other national advisory groups support consumption of diets rich in fruits and vegetables, lean proteins—including fish, skinless poultry, low-fat and nonfat dairy products—and fiber-rich grains. And a diet that's good for the heart is also good for the brain, digestive tract, and your waistline! There's plenty of choice and no deprivation.

# FOOD GROUPS THAT CAN INFLUENCE BLOOD CHOLESTEROL LEVELS

Foods to choose to help lower blood cholesterol levels:
- Fruits and vegetables
- Fish (salmon, sardines, tuna, herring—all rich in omega-3-fats)
- Poultry (skinless)
- Oats and other whole grains (brown rice, bulgur, quinoa)
- Lean beef (cuts such as sirloin, round, flank) (*optional*)
- Low-fat or nonfat dairy (milk, yogurt, cheese)
- Vegetable oils (olive, safflower, sunflower, corn)

Foods to limit to help lower blood cholesterol levels:
- Fatty cuts of beef, pork, lamb
- Full-fat dairy (milk, yogurt, cheese)
- Butter
- Liver
- Eggs*
- Seafood* (shrimp or lobster)

(*Updated dietary guidelines now support moderate intake, not severe restrictions.)

You might find that six months of a dietary intervention is sufficient to lower your cholesterol levels to a healthful range. But that is not true for many people, and often, in addition to dietary modifications, a medication must be added. And if dietary changes do *not* lower your cholesterol levels, it's not your fault! Your liver is producing too much cholesterol for your body's needs, and you have no control over that process—it's connected to your body's metabolism and genes. When it comes to lowering blood cholesterol levels, limiting cholesterol-boosting foods, and cutting the body's production with a medication is often the optimal one-two punch needed for a healthy blood cholesterol profile.

If the time comes when you do need to add a medication, it's not a "get out of jail free" card that allows you to eat whatever you want. Maintaining a diet that limits your cholesterol and saturated fat intake can definitely contribute to maintaining your blood cholesterol levels, often enabling you to lower your medication dosage to keep your cholesterol levels in a healthy range. It's a big mistake to believe that cholesterol-lowering medications "protect" an individual from any impact an unhealthy diet can have on cholesterol levels. Remember, blood cholesterol levels come from both the diet and what your body produces. Maintaining a diet modest in cholesterol and saturated fat can mean that you need to take a lower dose of medication to keep blood cholesterol levels under control. And this can mean fewer or no side effects. For any prescription medication, the goal is to use the lowest effective dose, so why not work with—not against—your body when it comes to the treatment of high cholesterol.

And while this book focuses on food as the lifestyle contribution to blood cholesterol levels, it's important to point out that being physically active—as little as walking for 30 minutes every day—can certainly contribute to healthier cholesterol levels, especially in raising your HDL (the "good" cholesterol).

## *Medications That Lower Cholesterol*

When a healthy diet and lifestyle are not sufficient to lower the concentrations of cholesterol in your blood, safe and effective medications are available to help keep those levels from becoming dangerously high and exposing you to multiple health risks.

Medications act in one of two ways to lower blood cholesterol. First, they act on the intestines to block dietary cholesterol absorption into the body. Second, they act on the liver, either to slow its production of cholesterol or to increases its ability to "vacuum" cholesterol from the blood. In deciding which drug is right for you, and how much you should take, your doctor will monitor blood cholesterol levels regularly to make sure that the dosage you are given reduces blood cholesterol but still maintains it at a level that supports overall health. A delicate balance!

That's why *what you eat* can have a significant impact on how well cholesterol-lowering medications work. Certain foods can either boost or reduce the impact of these medications on blood cholesterol levels.

There are *five* major categories of cholesterol-lowering drugs. Because each one acts differently to lower cholesterol, the foods to avoid when taking them also differ. If you use more than one medication, follow the food-medicine interaction guidelines for each of the drugs you take.

**TYPES OF CHOLESTEROL-LOWERING DRUGS:**

- Statins
- Bile acid binding drugs
- Fibric acid drugs
- Niacin
- Cholesterol absorption inhibitors

## Statins

Statins reduce blood cholesterol levels by reducing cholesterol production in the liver. Your liver produces less cholesterol, so less is released into the bloodstream. As a result, total cholesterol levels drop, as does your LDL cholesterol. This type of cholesterol is "bad" because it transports cholesterol to blood vessels, where it can clog them up. Sometimes, certain statin medications can *raise* the blood concentration of HDL cholesterol. This type of cholesterol is healthy because it picks up cholesterol throughout the blood stream and transports it to the liver for disposal. In this case, raising a cholesterol level is a good thing!

There are seven statin medications approved for use in the United States (see box).

### SEVEN STATIN MEDICATIONS USED TO LOWER CHOLESTEROL

- Atorvastatin (Lipitor®)
- Fluvastatin (Lescol®)
- Lovastatin (Mevacor)
- Pitavastatin (Livalo®)
- Pravastatin (Pravachol®)
- Rosuvastatin (Crestor®)
- Simvastatin (Zocor®; Vytorin® [a combination of simvastatin and ezetimibe])

Solid scientific research documents the association between being in the healthful blood cholesterol range and having a lower risk of developing heart disease. This applies to both healthy people with cardiovascular risk factors, and to people who already have a history of cardiovascular disease and are working at preventing a recurrence. These diseases include coronary artery disease, heart attack, stroke, or peripheral arterial disease.

For millions of people, using statin medications has become part of a major treatment plan for both prevention and recurrence of cardiovascular disease.

## *Foods to Avoid When Taking Statin Medications*

### Grapefruit

The best scientific studies on the important food interactions when taking the statin drugs focus on grapefruit and grapefruit juice.

Grapefruit naturally contains compounds that *inactivate* an important enzyme that breaks down certain statin drugs as they are absorbed from the intestines. When a statin is taken by mouth, it passes through the stomach and into the intestines. The cells in the intestine contain an enzyme that breaks down some of the statin as it is absorbed and passed into the circulation.

But when a statin pill is ingested by someone who consumes grapefruit or grapefruit juice, this enzyme doesn't do its job, more of the statin is absorbed, and blood levels of the statin may rise to much higher levels than occur in individuals who do not consume grapefruit. And higher blood levels of the statin may increase the likelihood of experiencing negative side effects of the statin medication—most commonly muscle pain and soreness.

Yet only *some* statins are vulnerable to this action of grapefruit: lovastatin (Mevacor), simvastatin (Zocor; or Vytorin [a combination of simvastatin and ezetimibe]), and, to a smaller extent, atorvastatin (Lipitor), since they are metabolized by the intestinal enzyme that is blocked by grapefruit. And if the enzyme breaking down the statin is blocked by grapefruit consumption, then more of the drug is absorbed into the bloodstream.

The good news is that some statins are not at all affected by grapefruit. But, when it comes to grapefruit, you must be quite sure which statin you are taking! As mentioned above, the three statins most definitely affected by grapefruit are lovastatin, simvastatin, and atorvastatin. If you're a grapefruit lover and take one of these three medicines, scientific data suggest it might *not* be harmful to consume limited amounts of grape- fruit—up to one serving daily of grapefruit (one-half) or grapefruit juice (6–8 ounces) a day. While this might seem confusing, it's really a matter of how much grape- fruit you eat each day—a little is OK (the enzyme is not affected), a lot is *not* OK (the enzyme is inhibited). If you are taking any of these three statins, talk to your doctor for personalized advice about your diet, and, if you are a grapefruit lover, whether you should switch to a statin that is not affected by grapefruit.

Also, since the compounds in grapefruit can con- tinue to affect the digestive enzyme for several days after you stop consuming grapefruit or grapefruit juice, if you are prescribed one of the statins that is sensitive to grapefruit (lovastatin, simvastatin, ator- vastatin), you should stop consuming grapefruit prod- ucts for about a week before you start taking one of these statins.

━━ If you are a grapefruit lover, and your doctor prescribes a statin drug for you, discuss the grapefruit issue carefully to make sure you have the appropriate medication and dietary strategy.

## Other Citrus Fruits

Two other citrus fruits—pomelos and Seville oranges—contain the same natural components of grapefruit that prevent the normal breakdown of the three statin drugs already mentioned (atorvastatin, lovastatin, simvastatin). A pomelo is a large Asian citrus fruit originally crossed with oranges to create a type of grapefruit. It is widely available in the United States and looks like a grapefruit. While most oranges do *not* typically contain the problematic components of grapefruit that inhibit statin effectiveness, Seville oranges are an exception. With consumption of pomelos or Seville oranges by people taking atorvastatin, lovastatin, or simvastatin, blood levels of the medication may rise to much higher levels than in individuals who do not consume them and increase the likelihood of side effects.

### AVOID GRAPEFRUIT, POMELO, AND SEVILLE ORANGES WHEN USING THESE STATINS

- Atorvastatin
- Lovastatin
- Simvastatin (Zocor, Vytorin)

## DIETARY SUPPLEMENT ALERT!

### Avoid St. John's Wort with Some Statins

The popular herbal supplement St. John's wort contains compounds that stimulate the breakdown of some statin drugs in the body, reducing their ability to lower serum cholesterol. Both simvastatin (Zocor, Vytorin) and atorvastatin (Lipitor) are known to be affected by St. John's wort. This means that, if you take St. John's wort and use either drug, your body would have *less* medication available than expected from your dose. Pravastatin (Pravachol), on the other hand, is not affected by using St. John's wort. As for the other statins, no information is available on whether St. John's wort is safe to take along with them.

It is essential to speak to your doctor if you currently use St. John's wort and are prescribed a statin, so that an appropriate medication can be chosen for you that is not affected by St. John's wort. And if you are already taking a statin, and do not use St. John's wort, but decide at some point to try this herbal supplement, talk to your doctor *before you do so*.

## DIETARY SUPPLEMENT ALERT!

### Red Yeast Rice with Statins

Red yeast rice *naturally* contains lovastatin (Mevacor), but in highly varying amounts. While sometimes used by consumers as an over-the-counter solution to treat elevated cholesterol, it is not regulated by the government for the amount of lovastatin it contains or for its purity and safety, as the prescription medication is. Taking a supplement of red yeast rice together with a statin drug may increase the risk of side effects like myopathy (muscle pain).

## *Bile Acid Binding Drugs*

Bile acid binding medicines (also known as sequestrant drugs) are *not* absorbed into the body but instead remain in the digestive tract after ingestion, ultimately leaving the body in the feces. As they pass through the intestines, they bind very tightly to compounds called "bile acids," and carry them out of the body. Bile acids are made in the liver from cholesterol and released into the intestines to help with dietary fat digestion and absorption in the digestive tract. Normally, bile acids are reabsorbed by the intestines after fat absorption and then reused. But when they are not reabsorbed, such as when a sequestrant drug is taken, the liver must make more to meet the body's needs. Since bile acids are formed from cholesterol, when the liver needs to produce more of them, more cholesterol is needed—which is removed from the bloodstream for this purpose. This results in lower blood cholesterol levels (primarily "bad" cholesterol, LDL).

Presently in the United States, three bile acid binding drugs are approved for use: cholestyramine (Questran®, Prevalite®), colesevelam (Welchol®), and colestipol (Colestid®). Currently, there are no important effects of foods on the ability of these drugs to act in the body. However, there *is* an important effect of these drugs on the absorption of some vitamins. Of particular concern is that these drugs may reduce the absorption of some of the fat-soluble vitamins (A, D, E, and K) and also the water-soluble vitamin folic acid. Folic acid is important to nervous system function, and, in pregnant women, folic acid deficiency can cause neural tube defects during fetal development.

If you are prescribed a bile acid binding medication, discuss with your doctor whether you should take a vitamin supplement to ensure adequate intakes of fat-soluble vitamins and folic acid (particularly if you are pregnant).

## *Fibric Acid Drugs*

The fibric acid drugs presently in use in the United States are gemfibrozil (Lopid®) and fenofibrate (Tricor®, Triglide®, Lofibra®, Antara®). These drugs are particularly useful for individuals with certain genetic disorders of fat metabolism that cause plasma lipid and cholesterol levels to be excessively high. Fibric acid drugs lower blood cholesterol and lipids through multiple metabolic actions on the liver and fat cells that promote the removal of cholesterol from the blood.

Consuming fibric acid medications with food can affect the availability of the drug to the blood. Food effects occur for gemfibrozil, and can occur for fenofibrate. There are *no* specific foods to be avoided—they just should not be taken at the same time you are eating.

---

If you are prescribed a fibric acid medication, discuss with your doctor the best time to take the drug in relation to meals and snacks.

---

## *Nicotinic Acid (Niacin)*

Nicotinic acid is a form of vitamin B2 (also called "niacin"). The vitamin B2 requirement in adults is quite low, around 15 mg daily. More than adequate amounts are usually found in the typical diet. Niacin is also found in most multivitamins in amounts meeting the daily requirement. Nicotinic acid is important in numerous reactions in the body, some of which are related to fat synthesis, storage, and metabolism.

Nicotinic acid is sometimes given to patients in amounts vastly greater than the daily requirement for good health. Taking very high daily doses of Niacin affects blood cholesterol levels in a similar way as statin drugs: it lowers the blood levels of the "lousy" LDL cholesterol and triglycerides, and raises blood levels of the "healthy" HDL cholesterol. Typical daily doses of niacin are 2 or more grams daily (2,000 or more mg daily), which is equal to at least 100 times the daily amount required for good health.

The use of nicotinic acid to treat high cholesterol levels is limited by its side effects, which are quite annoying. The vitamin causes severe flushing of the face and stomach upset, even at doses only modestly above daily nutritional requirements. Currently, the only known negative interaction with niacin occurs with the use of alcoholic beverages, which can increase flushing.

■ If your physician prescribes nicotinic acid (niacin) for you, discuss the side effects associated with this drug and whether you need to restrict alcohol intake below standard health recommendations (up to one serving a day for women; up to two servings per day for men).

## *Cholesterol Absorption Inhibitors*

Ezetimibe (Zetia) prevents dietary cholesterol from being absorbed from the intestines. As a result, cholesterol goes through the digestive track and is eliminated in the feces. This causes less cholesterol to be delivered into the bloodstream and lowers blood cholesterol levels. However, the liver senses this reduction and adjusts by making more cholesterol, which would seem to cancel out the effect of the drug. For this reason, ezetimibe is most often used in combination with a statin drug, which is used to block cholesterol formation in the liver. It's another example of that one-two punch to lower cholesterol levels in blood: prevent the liver from making cholesterol while blocking some dietary cholesterol from being absorbed by the body.

There are no known effects of nutrients or food on the action of ezetimibe; it is not known to influence the absorption of any nutrients, vitamins, or minerals into the body, except for cholesterol.

There are no known food interactions with a cholesterol absorption inhibitor.

## PATIENT STORY: JOAN

Joan had a family history of heart disease and went for a yearly physical with her primary care doctor. She learned that her fasting cholesterol had become elevated over the past year. Joan had gained about 15 pounds, and she was surprised to see that her total cholesterol had climbed to about 250, and her LDL had inched up into the 130–140 range.

She had also been trying to boost her dietary calcium intake, and mentioned to her doctor that she'd been adding a few ounces of cheddar cheese to her daily diet. (She was an admitted cheese lover!) Joan didn't recall any other major dietary changes over the past year. Her doctor first "prescribed" dietary changes to see if that might have sufficient impact. After all, her cholesterol levels were not dangerously elevated, and Joan was willing and able to make some changes in her eating habits. And so began her six-month revised eating plan.

She first cut back on her saturated fat intake and switched to nonfat milk and other dairy products. She decided she'd get added dietary calcium from nonfat plain yogurt, and eliminated her cheese. Joan's focus was to still eat a variety of foods, but limit her portions, to trim about 300–500 calories out during the day. This produced a rate of weight loss of about 0.5–1 pound a week. At the end of six months, Joan had lost about 12 pounds, and her cholesterol levels had dropped some, but not enough, her doctor said, to put her in the healthy range for both total and LDL cholesterol. He was proud of her lifestyle effort and explained that, because her dietary changes already produced some reduction in her cholesterol, he was optimistic that she would be able to stay on a low dose of medication, a big plus when it comes to minimizing possible side effects. Joan began a low dose of simvastatin (Zocor), and repeated blood testing showed her cholesterol to have decreased to a normal level for good health. Joan remained compliant with her diet and, along with taking a modest dose of statin, has managed her cholesterol very well. Both Joan and her doctor are very pleased with her health.

## PATIENT STORY: JOHN

At age 35, John was surprised when his doctor suggested that taking a statin would be a good idea. According to his doctor, his total cholesterol level was elevated, despite decreasing his saturated fat intake over the past six months. His BMI was elevated, placing him in the overweight category, but he was a healthy eater and enjoyed outdoor activities, such as gardening and yard work. However, he did have several family members already taking statins, and both his father and grandfather had cardiovascular disease. He figured statins were worth a try but was concerned about the side effects he'd heard about from his family.

John started on atorvastatin (Lipitor), which lowered his cholesterol to mid-range, considered normal by the cholesterol guidelines, but he began to have muscle aches in his legs. Two of his cousins also had this side effect. While atorvastatin was covered by his insurance, some other medications were not. John spoke with his doctor and agreed that a statin was a health plus, but asked if he could switch to another drug that wouldn't give him leg pain. His doctor suggested rosuvastatin (Crestor), another statin that often is used in lower doses with the same effectiveness. Happily, switching to rosuvastatin worked for him, and his only decision was a financial one. John's health insurance had a higher co-pay for rosuvastatin, but he felt that the benefits far outweighed the extra out-of-pocket expenses.

# Chapter 8
# HEART (Cardiovascular) MEDICINES

Your heart is the hardest-working muscle in the whole body. It beats regularly 24/7; most of us take this activity for granted and don't even pay attention to the steady beat. However, the heart pumps blood throughout the body, which supplies nutrients to every cell in the body, and carries away waste products produced by normal cellular activity. The system of blood vessels both going into and leaving the heart is a complex and awesome structure.

While we assume our hearts will always be working as designed, for millions of people, the heart as a pump can develop several different kinds of problems that reduce its ability to function effectively. When heart function is impaired, medication is often used to boost and help normalize it.

Heart problems arise in two main ways: the heart muscle itself is damaged or weakened (as in a heart attack); or the heartbeat becomes abnormal, and beats too fast, too slow, or in an irregular way—changes that are not healthy for the body. In both cases, your heart becomes inefficient at pumping blood through the arteries. The blood leaves the heart rich in oxygen, and is pumped through the arteries to all parts of the body. When the heart cannot pump the blood into the arteries effectively, all body organs are at risk of damage. There is a group of very effective medications to stabilize these problems and help restore heart function to as close to normal as possible.

Just as the heart needs to pump blood to the entire body, it also pumps it to itself through small arteries that travel throughout the heart muscle. If the blood supply into the heart muscle slows down, a very uncomfortable feeling in your chest can result, called "angina," which is short for the medical term "angina pectoris." The tightness and discomfort in your chest caused by angina usually indicates that the heart muscle is not getting enough blood (known in medical terms as "ischemia"), which is bad for heart function. The good news is that there are effective medicines that control the cause of angina and support healthy heart function.

While this chapter examines heart drugs, a discussion of certain lung ailments must also be addressed. The connection and relationship between your heart and your lungs is intimate; both work closely together. So in this chapter, we'll also talk about a special type of high blood pressure called "primary pulmonary hypertension" that affects heart function. This particular type of high blood pressure occurs in the large blood vessel (the pulmonary artery) that carries blood the very short distance from the heart to the lungs.

## HEART AILMENTS REQUIRING MEDICATIONS

- Angina (an uncomfortable feeling in the chest area indicating inadequate blood flow to heart muscle)
- Heart arrhythmias (abnormal beating of the heart)
- Congestive heart failure (heart muscle function impaired)
- Primary pulmonary hypertension (heart-lung circulation impaired)

## *Drugs Used to Treat Angina (Inadequate Blood Flow to Heart Muscle)*

Among the most common of heart ailments, angina is a very uncomfortable feeling of pressure or tightening over the chest, sometimes accompanied by pain. This discomfort reflects insufficient blood flowing into the heart muscle to support its energy needs. When blood flow into the heart muscle is too slow, the heart uses oxygen faster than it can be supplied, and then runs out of it! Without enough oxygen, the heart cannot function normally for very long. The good news is that there are effective drugs to increase blood flow into the heart muscle that act almost immediately after you take them. These medications act by relaxing the arteries going into the heart muscle. As a result, the blood vessels open up, actually becoming wider, enabling more blood (and oxygen) to flow into the heart muscle.

Organic nitrates (nitroglycerin, for example) make up a main class of drugs that relax the blood vessels going into the heart muscle. These nitrates are the focus of this chapter. Two other types of medications, "calcium channel blockers" and "beta blockers," are also effective for angina, but work in a different way from organic nitrates. If you take these medications for angina, see chapter 6 (blood pressure medicines) for a discussion of food and supplement interactions with them. Even statins and antiplatelet medications can be used in the treatment of angina. Refer to chapter 7 for a discussion of statin medications, and chapter 3 for a discussion of antiplatelet medicines concerning food and supplement interactions.

## MEDICATIONS USED FOR THE TREATMENT OF ANGINA

Organic nitrates:
- Nitroglycerin (Minitran®, Nitro-Bid®, Nitro-Dur®, Nitro-Time®, Nitrolingual®, NitroMist®, Nitrostat®, Rectiv®)
- Isosorbide (isosorbide dinitrate— Isordil®, Dilatrate-SR®; isosorbide mononitrate— Imdur®)
- Ranolazine (Ranexa®)

Other related drug categories:
- Calcium channel blockers and beta blockers (see chapter 6)
- Antiplatelet drugs (see chapter 3)
- Statins (see chapter 7)

It's important to avoid alcoholic beverages when taking nitroglycerin or isosorbide drugs. These drugs dilate (open up) blood vessels to boost blood flow into the heart muscle, but they also dilate *all* blood vessels in the body, which causes blood pressure to fall. As a result, a common side effect of these drugs is dizziness and faintness when you stand up. Alcohol also dilates blood vessels, so the dizziness or faintness may increase if you are taking an organic nitrite drug and consume an alcoholic beverage. The safety of drinking alcoholic beverages while you are under treatment with these medicines is an important issue that you should discuss with your doctor.

**FOODS TO AVOID WHEN TAKING
NITROGLYCERIN OR ISOCARBIDE
MEDICATIONS FOR ANGINA**

Alcoholic beverages

Many herbal supplements can also cause reductions in blood pressure—making them risky to take when you are using organic nitrates. These include coenzyme Q10, Asian ginseng, hawthorn, and melatonin. Hawthorn may also increase blood flow to heart muscle, potentially adding to the effect of the drug you are taking. A large variety of herbal supplements can reduce blood pressure, and some may also affect blood flow to heart muscle. For this reason, it's very important for you to discuss your use of herbal supplements if your doctor has asked you to take a drug for angina. We're limiting our discussion here to the "top 10" supplements, so if you don't see your dietary supplement on our list, please make sure to check out one of these excellent online sources of information for your specific supplement: WebMD (webmd.com), Drugs.com, the Office of Dietary Supplements (ods. od.nih.gov/factsheets/list-all), or the National Center for Complementary and Integrative Health (nccih. nih.gov/health/herbsataglance.htm) at the National Institutes of Health.

And avoid using St. John's wort when taking isosorbide. St. John's wort reduces the availability of this medication to your body, making the prescribed dose *less* effective.

**DIETARY SUPPLEMENT ALERT!**

**Avoid These Supplements When Taking Nitroglycerin or Isosorbide Medications for Angina:**

Coenzyme Q10
Asian Ginseng
Hawthorn
Melatonin
St. John's wort (if taking isosorbide)
*Any* supplement that claims to lower blood pressure or treat angina

Another type of medication used to treat angina and impaired blood flow to the heart muscle is ranolazine (Ranexa). If you take this drug, avoid St. John's wort, because it reduces the effectiveness of the drug. And avoid grapefruit and grapefruit juice, because they increase the effectiveness of the drug, so side effects may be greater (such as feeling faint).

## *Drugs Used to Treat Irregular Heartbeat (Arrhythmias)*

Experiencing abnormal beating of your heart is very scary. Your heart might beat too fast, too slow, or unevenly (a feeling like you "skipped a beat"). These kinds of changes in your heartbeat can cause palpitations, breathlessness, dizziness, or fainting—as well as more serious consequences, including a heart attack. The good news is that very effective medications are available to stabilize your heartbeat and support normal cardiac function. The drugs that do this are called anti-arrhythmics, or medicines that reduce irregular heartbeats.

You'll work closely with your doctor to determine which drug and dose is most effective. The dosage must be determined very carefully, because it doesn't take much more medicine above the optimal dose to cause negative side effects. This means that, when you're taking one of these drugs, you need to be especially careful to *avoid* food and dietary supplements that can boost the effects of the drug. And because paying attention to the potential interference of certain foods and dietary supplements is a key to success in using these medications, and advice on this can vary from drug to drug, we discuss each anti-arrhythmia drug separately to be clear.

## FOODS TO AVOID WITH ANTI-ARRHYTHMIA MEDICATIONS

*Note:* With all the drugs listed below, be consistent in taking them with or without food.

With amiodarone (Cordarone®, Pacerone®):
- Grapefruit and grapefruit juice

With dronedarone (Multaq®):
- Grapefruit and grapefruit juice

With disopyramide (Norpace®, Norpace CR®):
- Grapefruit and grapefruit juice

With quinidine (Gluconate® or Sulfate form):
- Limit all fruit juices
- Limit citrus fruits, especially grapefruit
- Limit foods containing vitamin C
- Keep salt intake consistent daily
- Limit calcium (dairy products, antacids, supplements)

With sotalol (Betapace®, Sorine®):
- Do not mix with calcium-containing foods (dairy, antacids, calcium supplements)—allow two or more hours before consuming these foods
- Limit alcohol intake

With dofetilide (Tikosyn®):
- Limit intake of grapefruit and grapefruit juice
- Consume a potassium and magnesium rich diet

With flecainide (Tambocor®):
- No specific foods to avoid or limit

With propafenone (Rythmol®):
- No specific foods to avoid or limit

## Amiodarone and Dronedarone

Amiodarone (Cordarone; Pacerone) and dronedarone (Multaq) can be taken with or without food. And the important point is to choose one way and stick with it. That's because food (especially fat-containing food) increases their absorption into blood. To avoid any variation in the drug's absorption and effects on the body, these drugs *must be taken consistently every day*, either with food or without food. Remember that taking these drugs with food translates into your body seeing *more* drug. If you take it on an empty stomach, your body would see *less* drug. This is an important issue when discussing appropriate dosage with your doctor.

Grapefruit and grapefruit juice also make more drug available to the body when you take it. So it becomes important to *avoid grapefruit or grapefruit juice* while you are taking either of these drugs.

You also need to avoid St. John's wort while taking these drugs, as this herbal supplement reduces drug absorption. This translates into your body seeing a lower dose of the medication than your doctor intended, which can impair its ability to control the arrhythmia.

## Disopyramide

Disopyramide (Norpace; Norpace CR) is a medication that can be taken without regard to food. The effect of the drug is the same whether you take it with or without food. It is important to avoid consuming grapefruit or grapefruit juice while taking this medicine, because grapefruit products can boost the action of the medication in the body. This translates into your body seeing a higher dose of the medication than your doctor intended.

There's an important dietary supplement alert for this medicine: *do not use St. John's wort!* Use of this herbal supplement will cause the blood level of the drug to be *lower*, translating into your body seeing a *lower* dose of the medication than intended. You might not have a sufficient amount of the medication to control your symptoms.

## Quinidine (Gluconate or Sulfate Forms)

Quinidine (gluconate or sulfate forms) can be taken with or without food. Importantly, food *can* affect drug absorption, so it is most important to be consistent from day to day in your habits. *Choose to take this medicine either with or without food, but the same way every day.* This medication has certain food issues that alter the availability (and effects) of this drug in your body. Salt in food can reduce drug absorption, so be consistent in your use of salt from day to day. For people with heart disease, The American Heart Association recommends keeping your total intake of sodium at 1,500 mg or less every day. Remember that packaged and processed foods usually contain higher sodium than fresh foods, so read the nutrition information on labels carefully.

Limit your intake of vitamin C (ascorbate, ascorbic acid) and fruit juices containing vitamin C (citrus juices contain the most), because they lower drug levels in blood (by increasing elimination in the urine). From the nutritional perspective, your body needs no more than about 100 mg a day, which is about the amount in 8 ounces of orange juice (or a multivitamin). If you take a vitamin C supplement, you are likely taking much more than this, and you should cut back if you are taking quinidine.

Avoid grapefruit and grapefruit juice, as grapefruit increases the bioavailability of this drug in the body.

Limit calcium intake from all sources. This means monitor your intake of dairy products (milk, yogurt, cheese), antacids (that contain calcium), and calcium supplements of all types. Calcium can raise drug levels in the blood (by reducing their breakdown and elimination from the body). The dietary requirement for calcium is around 1,000 mg each day, so take stock of your calcium intake and stay as close to the requirement amount as possible.

As with other anti-arrhythmia medications, avoid St. John's wort. This herbal supplement reduces the level of medication circulating in your bloodstream, which your body sees as a lower dose of the medication. It's not what your doctor intended and can modify the effectiveness of the medicine in treating your symptoms.

## Sotalol

Sotalol (Betapace, Sorine) must be taken consistently either with or without food. This is important because the absorption of the medication is reduced when taken with food, translating into a lower dose seen by your body over time. It's also important not to take foods, supplements or antacids containing calcium, magnesium or aluminum at the same time you take this medication. Take your drug two hours or more before you ingest any such products. This includes calcium-rich dairy products: take your medication at least two hours before you consume any dairy foods. The concern is that these minerals bind to the medication in the stomach and intestines, preventing its absorption into the bloodstream. This *reduces* the beneficial actions of the medicine.

Sotalol makes your heartbeat more regular, but it also lowers blood pressure. Since this medication reduces your blood pressure, it is essential to limit your intake of alcoholic beverages while using this drug. The combination of alcohol with the medication can cause a bigger drop in blood pressure than when the drug is taken alone. As a result, you might feel light-headed or dizzy.

Herbal supplements that lower blood pressure should also be avoided. If you use any herbal supplements to lower blood pressure, they may enhance the blood pressure-lowering effect of sotalol and make you dizzy and light-headed. Some of these supplements are listed on pages 135–138, along with referrals to websites that allow you to identify others that may lower blood pressure. If you use any of these or other herbal supplements that claim to lower blood pressure, it is advisable to discontinue their use while taking sotalol.

## Dofetilide

Dofetilide (Tikosyn) can be taken with or without food. The only food concern is a possible effect of grapefruit and grapefruit juice. Grapefruit may cause a small increase in the availability of dofetilide in the body. For this reason, if you consume grapefruit or grapefruit juice, it is advisable to limit your daily intake to half a grapefruit or a small glass of grapefruit juice (6–8 ounces).

Because of how dofetilide acts on the heart, it is important to consume adequate amounts of both potassium and magnesium in your diet. Your doctor should monitor your blood levels of these electrolytes and, if low, encourage you to consume more foods that contain significant amounts of them (see Table 3 for examples of potassium-rich foods and Table 4 for magnesium-rich foods). With monitoring, your doctor can determine if your dietary intake of these minerals is sufficient, or whether a supplement might be needed while you are taking this medication.

## TABLE 3. POTASSIUM-RICH FOODS

(Aim for at least 4,700 mg/day.)

| Food | Amount | mg |
|---|---|---|
| Winter squash | 1 cup cubed | 900 |
| Sweet potato | medium (with skin) | 690 |
| White potato (with skin) | medium (with skin) | 610 |
| Yogurt | 1 cup | 580 |
| Halibut | 3 ounces cooked | 490 |
| 100% orange juice | 1 cup | 500 |
| Broccoli | 1 cup | 460 |
| Cantaloupe | 1 cup cubed | 430 |
| Banana | 1 medium | 420 |
| Pork tenderloin | 3 ounces cooked | 380 |
| Lentils | ½ cup | 270 |
| Milk | 8 ounces | 370 |
| Salmon | 3 ounces cooked | 325 |
| Pistachio nuts | 1 ounce shelled | 295 |

## TABLE 4. MAGNESIUM-RICH FOODS

(Aim for more than 300 mg/day [women];
more than 400 mg/day [men].)

| Food | Amount | Magnesium (mg) |
|---|---|---|
| Dark-green, leafy vegetables | 1 cup | 160 |
| Soy beans | 1 cup | 70 |
| Black beans | 1 cup | 120 |
| Almonds | 1 ounce | 75 |
| Cashews | 1 ounce | 85 |
| Banana | 1 medium | 30 |
| Oatmeal | 1 cup | 60 |
| Quinoa | ½ cup | 120 |
| Lentils | 1 cup | 70 |
| Brown rice | 1 cup | 85 |
| Whole wheat bread | 2 slices | 45 |

Flecainide (Tambocor) and propafenone (Rythmol) can be taken with or without food. One special case applies to flecainide: it is approved for use in infants and, when prescribed, should *not* be given at the same time as dairy products (milk or milk-based infant formulas), as absorption of the drug may be reduced. This means that the drug's effects may also be reduced and appear to the body as a lower dose. If your infant is taking this medication, make sure to ask your doctor about the best timing of drug administration in relation to feedings of milk-based food products.

---

**DIETARY SUPPLEMENT ALERT!**

**Avoid When Taking Anti-Arrhythmia Medications:**

St. John's wort:
- Amiodarone (Cordarone, Pacerone)
- Dronedarone (Multaq)
- Disopyramide (Norpace; Norpace CR)
- Quinidine (gluconate or sulfate form)

Supplements that may lower blood pressure (see pages 135–138 for list of commonly used products):
- Sotalol (Betapace; Sorine)

---

## *Digoxin for the Treatment of Congestive Heart Failure*

Congestive heart failure takes many years to develop. It is characterized by the inability of the heart to pump enough blood to meet the needs of all of the organs of the body. This can occur for many reasons and treatment usually involves a sequence of different drugs.

Many drugs that treat high blood pressure are used at various stages of heart disease, as heart failure develops. If you're taking an antihypertensive medication as part of your heart failure drug plan, read chapter 6 to learn about food and medicine interactions involving those medications.

The one drug used *only* for the treatment of heart failure—digoxin (Lanoxin®)—is discussed here.

Digoxin (Lanoxin) increases the strength of the heartbeat. This results in a greater amount of blood entering the arteries and increased blood flow throughout the body. The blood circulating from the arteries provides nutrients and oxygen to all body tissues, so a boost in the flow of blood into the arteries is essential to normal organ and body function.

You can take digoxin with or without food—with one big exception: you should not consume the drug along with foods and meals that are high in dietary fiber, including foods high in pectin, a type of fiber. When fiber is consumed with digoxin, the absorption of the drug into the blood is greatly reduced, as is the beneficial effect on the heart.

Pectin is present in many foods. There are high amounts of pectin in fruits (apricots, peaches, apples, oranges), vegetables (carrots, peas, potatoes, tomatoes), and cereals (cornflakes). If you consume large amounts of fiber in your diet, you should tell your doctor and discuss the best strategy to maintain a healthy diet to optimize the action of the drug. You can avoid the problem entirely by taking digoxin a few hours *before* meals. But upon your doctor's recommendation, you may need to reduce the total amount of daily dietary fiber you consume.

The ingestion of grapefruit and grapefruit juice can cause digoxin levels in blood to rise, while ingestion of St. John's wort can cause them to fall. The aluminum present in some common antacids inhibits absorption of the drug and thus reduces blood digoxin levels if the two are taken together. These items should probably be avoided while you are taking this drug, as even small changes in blood digoxin levels can alter the drug's beneficial effects on the heart (as well as the occurrence of side effects).

---

**FOODS TO AVOID WHEN TAKING DIGOXIN**

- Fiber-rich foods

- Pectin-rich foods (apricots, peaches, apples, oranges, carrots, peas, potatoes, tomatoes)

- Grapefruit and grapefruit juice

- Antacids containing aluminum (not a food, but an over-the-counter product)

---

## *Drugs Used to Treat Primary Pulmonary Hypertension*

To understand what primary pulmonary hypertension actually means requires a short and easy anatomy lesson. The heart functions as a pump that pushes blood through one set of blood vessels into the lungs, receives it back from the lungs, and then sends it out through another set of vessels to supply all of the other parts of the body. The assembly of vessels sending blood to and from the lungs is the *pulmonary circulation* (pulmonary means lungs), while the network of vessels sending blood to and from all of the other parts of the body is the *systemic circulation*. As you know, the lungs are a specialized organ that supplies oxygen to the blood and removes carbon dioxide, a "waste" gas. The other parts of the body remove the oxygen from blood, use it to generate energy, and return to it carbon dioxide, the waste gas generated from the use of oxygen. Overall, the lungs provide oxygen to the blood for the other parts of the body to use, which they do, and in the process generate carbon dioxide that they release back into blood, which is sent back to the lungs to be eliminated.

The heart sends blood into the systemic circulation at a sufficiently high pressure to ensure that blood can reach all the parts of the body served very quickly. In contrast, the heart sends the blood into the lungs at a very low pressure.

Why is blood pressure so low in the lungs? It's because the blood vessel walls in the lungs are extremely thin, permitting oxygen to move very quickly from the airways of the lungs into the blood, and for carbon dioxide to move very quickly from blood into the airways. High pressure here can damage these vessels, causing leakage of blood and fluid into the lung airways. This sounds like a scary situation—and it is! It is life threatening because it makes breathing very difficult.

This is the condition that develops in primary pulmonary hypertension. Because it is a life-threatening condition, it must be treated. The drugs currently available in the United States to treat primary pulmonary hypertension are sildenafil (Revatio®) and tadalafil (Adcirca®).

## Sildenafil and Tadalafil

Both sildenafil (Revatio) and tadalafil (Adcirca) can be taken with or without food. You should avoid alcoholic beverages when taking these medications because they reduce blood pressure, and this effect is increased by alcohol ingestion. If your blood pressure drops too much, you could become dizzy and faint.

You should also avoid grapefruit and grapefruit juice, as they can cause the level of the drug in your blood to increase, which your body senses as a higher dose and can lead to unpleasant side effects.

It's essential to discontinue the dietary supplement St. John's wort because it can cause blood drug levels to fall, reducing the beneficial effects of these medications.

**MEDICATION AND FOOD INTERACTIONS WITH PRIMARY PULMONARY HYPERTENSION TREATMENT**

Medications used to treat primary pulmonary hypertension:
- Sildenafil (Revatio)
- Tadalafil (Adcirca)

Foods to avoid when taking primary pulmonary hypertension drugs:
- Grapefruit and grapefruit juice
- Alcohol

**DIETARY SUPPLEMENT ALERT!**

**Avoid Taking with Primary Pulmonary Hypertension Drugs:**

St. John's wort

## PATIENT STORY: SAM

Sam, now in his mid-50s, had a strong family history of heart disease and opted for preventive care for his heart, beginning in his 30s. While he did have a minor heart attack in his 40s, his doctor told him the damage to his heart was minimal, and he was able to resume his healthy lifestyle activities over time. He managed his weight well, was a healthy eater, and took a daily walk. Even with a healthy lifestyle, he needed some medication to help moderate his blood pressure.

Over the years, he was very attuned to changes in his body and noticed regular episodes of feeling some tightness in his chest—not pain, but pressure, a discomfort. He immediately went to his cardiologist for a consultation, where he was diagnosed with mild angina, and his doctor prescribed nitroglycerin tablets to place under his tongue when needed. Sam wasn't happy to take an additional medication but was relieved to have a diagnosis, and a medication that could support his own optimal heart function.

All went well for a few weeks, but Sam noticed from time to time that, when he used his nitroglycerin, he felt dizzy and nauseous and got a terrific headache. He couldn't figure out why. He wondered if the medication was too strong for him. His cardiologist identified the problem on Sam's next visit. Sam enjoyed a daily glass of red wine; he had added it as a health boost, on the advice of a friend. Since alcohol can enhance the effects of nitroglycerin, his doctor suggested eliminating the daily glass of red wine for a while to see if this affected the treatment. The interaction of the alcohol with his medication turned out to be the problem, so Sam discontinued his daily glass of red wine. Happily, his symptoms went away and did not return. Now Sam chooses a glass of seltzer with a splash of cranberry juice and a lime instead of any alcoholic beverage. He finds this works well in social situations as well as at home.

## PATIENT STORY: TERRI

Terri had struggled with chronic heart disease for many years. Now in her mid-60s, she'd had coronary artery bypass surgery about a decade ago. This greatly improved her health, but she knew her heart was losing strength. On the positive side, she followed all of her cardiologist's recommendations for a healthy lifestyle. She generally ate a plant-based protein diet (although she had a lean hamburger weekly with her girlfriends when they went out for lunch). Her diet was rich in fruits and vegetables, and she ate fiber-rich whole grains. On her most recent visit, she was told by her doctor that she needed to add digoxin to help boost the strength of her heart. While she was not pleased to add another drug to her regimen, Terri understood from earlier discussions that this would be a likely addition at some point.

Before starting Terri on this medication, her cardiologist asked about her diet. At first, that puzzled Terri, but she figured there might be a food or two she'd need to eliminate or modify. She had heard of food and medicine interactions. She was surprised to hear that one whole category of food—dietary fiber—could have a major impact on how digoxin worked in her body. Too much fiber reduced the absorption of digoxin, lowering its effect on her heart. Terri was concerned about how she would maintain a healthy diet without abundant fiber.

The solution was to take the digoxin in the mid-afternoon, because she was not a snacker. She always ate lunch at noon and dinner no earlier than 6:00 p.m. By taking her medication at 2:30 p.m. every day, she avoided the fiber issue completely—the medication would be absorbed when there was no fiber around. She could maintain her current healthy eating habits and not compromise the action of the digoxin.

# Resources

Websites with more information on dietary and herbal supplements:

- Drugs.com

- WebMD (webmd.com)

- National Center for Complementary and Integrative Health (nccih.nih.gov/health/herbsataglance.htm)

- Office of Dietary Supplements, National Institutes of Health (https://ods.od.nih.gov/factsheets/list-all/)

# Acknowledgments

We appreciate the support of our children, Aaron and Lauren, who were enthusiasts from the start, and have always been supportive of our creative and professional work together. Special thanks to Lauren, whose careful reading of the final manuscript along with her insightful suggestions were a big help to us.

We are most grateful for the medical editorial advice provided by Jeffrey G. Hirsch, MD (Madelyn's brother and John's brother-in-law). His thoughtful comments and suggestions were extremely helpful.

Many thanks to our publisher, Tony Lyons, who shared our passion for bringing this book to readers everywhere. We also very much appreciate the hard work on the manuscript from our senior editor, Krishan Trotman, and our copyeditor, Pam Owen.

# Index